Non-Visual Human-Computer Interactions
Prospects for the visually handicapped

Communication non visuelle homme-ordinateur
Perspectives pour les personnes handicapées de la vue

Colloques **INSERM**
ISSN 0768-3154

Other *Colloques* published as co-editions by John Libbey Eurotext and INSERM

133 Cardiovascular and Respiratory Physiology in the Fetus and Neonate. *Physiologie Cardiovasculaire et Respiratoire du Fœtus et du Nouveau-né.*
Scientific Committee : P. Karlberg,
A. Minkowski, W. Oh and L. Stern;
Managing Editor : M. Monset-Couchard.
ISBN : John Libbey Eurotext 0 86196 086 6
INSERM 2 85598 282 0

134 Porphyrins and Porphyrias. *Porphyrines et Porphyries.*
Edited by Y. Nordmann.
ISBN : John Libbey Eurotext 0 86196 087 4
INSERM 2 85598 281 2

137 Neo-Adjuvant Chemotherapy. *Chimiothérapie Néo-Adjuvante.*
Edited by C. Jacquillat, M. Weil and D. Khayat.
ISBN : John Libbey Eurotext 0 86196 077 7
INSERM 2 85598 283 7

139 Hormones and Cell Regulation (10th European Symposium). *Hormones et Régulation Cellulaire (10ᵉ Symposium Européen).*
Edited by J. Nunez, J.E. Dumont and R.J.B. King.
ISBN : John Libbey Eurotext 0 86196 084 X
INSERM 2 85598 284 7

147 Modern Trends in Aging Research. *Nouvelles Perspectives de la Recherche sur le Vieillissement.*
Edited by Y. Courtois, B. Faucheux, B. Forette, D.L. Knook and J.A. Tréton.
ISBN : John Libbey Eurotext 0 86196 103 X
INSERM 2 85598 309 6

149 Binding Proteins of Steroid Hormones. *Protéines de liaison des Hormones Stéroïdes.*
Edited by M.G. Forest and M. Pugeat.
ISBN : John Libbey Eurotext 0 86196 125 0
INSERM 2 85598 310 X

151 Control and Management of Parturition. *La Maîtrise de la Parturition.*
Edited by C. Sureau, P. Blot, D. Cabrol, F. Cavaillé and G. Germain.
ISBN : John Libbey Eurotext 0 86196 096 3
INSERM 2 85598 311 8

Suite page 207
(Continued p. 207)

Non-Visual Human-Computer Interactions
Prospects for the visually handicapped

Communication non visuelle homme-ordinateur
Perspectives pour les personnes handicapées de la vue

Proceedings of the INSERM-SETAA Conference
Ministère de la Recherche et de l'Espace
Paris, 29-30 March, 1993

Actes du Colloque INSERM-SETAA
Ministère de la Recherche et de l'Espace
Paris, 29-30 mars 1993

Under the patronage of :
Sous le patronage de :

Secrétariat d'Etat aux Handicapés et Accidentés de la Vie
Institut National de la Santé et de la Recherche Médicale
Département Homme-Travail-Technologie du Ministère
de la Recherche et de l'Espace

Edited by

Dominique Burger
Jean-Claude Sperandio

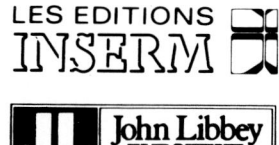

LES EDITIONS
INSERM

John Libbey
EUROTEXT

British Library Cataloguing in Publication Data
A catalogue record for this book
is available from the British Library

ISBN 2 7420 0014 3
ISSN 0768-3154

First published in 1993 by

Editions John Libbey Eurotext
6 rue Blanche, 92120 Montrouge, France. (33) (1) 47 35 85 52
ISBN 2 7420 0014 3

John Libbey and Company Ltd
13 Smiths Yard, Summerley Street, London SW18 4HR,
England.
(44) (81) 947 27 77

Institut National de la Santé et de la Recherche Médicale
101 rue de Tolbiac, 75654 Paris Cedex 13, France.
(33) (1) 44 23 60 00
ISBN 2 85 598 540 4

ISSN 0768-3154

© 1993 Colloques INSERM/John Libbey Eurotext Ltd,
All rights reserved
Unauthorized publication contravenes applicable laws

Foreword

Computers are becoming universal tools which help people access information, exchange messages, produce documents, images and even objects. They are also playing an increasingly important role in the learning process.

At the same time, because computers are expected to reach a large public, interfaces are becoming more intuitive. For instance, the generalization of metaphorical presentation styles has led to new interaction modalities such as speech and gesture, control, handwriting recognition and tactile and speech outputs.

This evolution clearly opens new outlooks for people who are unable to operate existing computers due to a physical or sensory limitation. In particular, the dialogue method based on the triad of the *keyboard, mouse* and *screen* which is highly dependent on vision, will soon be considered as just one possibility among others.

Thus, one major concern of these developments is the improvement of computer access for the visually handicapped.

Nevertheless, since these developments are quite recent and since they are probably still to come, it is not surprising that both theoretical and pragmatical references needed by computer scientists to create non-visual interfaces are still rather scarce.

On the occasion of this conference, specialists in the fields of cognition, education, ergonomics, computer sciences and neurosciences review elements of theory and present concrete experiences that seem to be particularly relevant to the discussion of prospects for non-visual human-computer interactions. Emphasis is placed on the following points:
– linguistic description of images,
– mental images in the blind,
– power of pictorial communication,
– object manipulation,
– multimodal human-computer interfaces,
– alternative access to existing software,
– tactile, auditory and verbal presentation of data.

Obviously, not all aspects of non-visual human-computer interactions can be covered in a two-day seminar.

It is nevertheless hoped that the work initiated here will be of some use to those interested in creating pluridisciplinary research projects aimed at developing *Non-visual human-computer interactions*.

Dominique Burger
Jean-Claude Sperandio

Préface

L'ordinateur est désormais un outil aux usages multiples grâce auquel il nous est possible d'accéder aux informations, d'échanger des messages, de mettre en forme et produire des documents, des images, mais également des objets matériels. L'ordinateur est également un moyen d'acquérir ou de transmettre des connaissances.

Parallèlement, son utilisation devient plus simple et intuitive. Pour répondre aux besoins d'un public de plus en plus large, les logiciels adoptent fréquemment un style de présentation métaphorique permettant, par exemple, de manipuler directement des objets à l'écran. Par ailleurs, de nouveaux modes d'interaction se développent, tels la commande vocale, le contrôle par le geste, la reconnaissance d'écriture manuscrite, les sorties vocales et tactiles.

Cette évolution ouvre de nouvelles perspectives pour les personnes à qui une incapacité physique ou sensorielle rend difficile l'accès aux applications de l'informatique. Les personnes handicapées de la vue sont particulièrement concernées puisque le dialogue reposant sur la triade *clavier-souris-écran,* largement dépendant de la vision, ne sera bientôt qu'une méthode parmi d'autres.

Cependant le développement de solutions adaptées, mettant en jeu de nouveaux modes d'interaction non visuels demande que soient mises en place des bases de connaissance nécessaires, en faisant appel aux différentes disciplines concernées.

L'objectif de cet ouvrage est d'amorcer ce travail en présentant des éléments théoriques et des réalisations concrètes dans le domaine des sciences cognitives, de l'éducation, de l'ergonomie, de l'informatique et des neurosciences. Les auteurs, spécialistes dans ces divers domaines, mettent en particulier l'accent sur les aspects suivants :
– description des images,
– images mentales chez l'aveugle,
– bases de la communication pictographique,
– manipulation des objets,
– interfaces multimodales,
– techniques d'accès aux applications logicielles,
– présentations tactile, auditive et verbale de données.

Il est clair que tous les aspects utiles à cette réflexion ne sauraient être couverts par un séminaire de deux jours. Nous espérons néanmoins que le travail original puisse être utile à tous ceux qui souhaitent participer à des projets de recherche et de développement visant l'amélioration de la *Communication non visuelle homme-ordinateur.*

Dominique Burger
Jean-Claude Sperandio

Scientific Committee
Comité scientifique

AYME Ségolène, INSERM France; BARKER Philip, University of Teeside, United Kingdom; BEROULE Dominique, CNRS, France; FLUHR Christian, INSTN-CEN, France; HATWELL Yvette, Université de Grenoble II, France; ROUSSEAU Alain, CNRS, France; STREMPEL Uli, Stiftung Blinden Anstalt Frankfurt, Germany

Organizing Committee
Comité d'organisation

BURGER Dominique, INSERM, France; SPERANDIO Jean-Claude, Université René-Descartes, France; GOLDBERG Marcel, INSERM, France; JOULIA Jean-Louis, SETAA-ANPEA, France; BURNOD Yves, INSERM, France.

The Conference was supported by
Le Colloque a reçu le soutien de

L'Institut National de la Santé et de la Recherche Médicale (INSERM)
Le Département Homme-Technologie-Travail du Ministère de la Recherche et de l'Espace
La Direction Scientifique de la DRET, Ministère de la Défense – DGA
L'Association nationale de Gestion de Fonds pour l'Insertion Professionnel des Handicapés (AGEFIPH)
L'Agence Nationale pour l'Amélioration des Conditions de Travail (ANACT)
Services et Techniques pour Aveugles et Amblyopes (SETAA)
Naturalia et Biologia (NEB)
L'Association Valentin Haüy pour le bien des aveugles (AVH)

Aknowledgements
Remerciements

We would like to express our gratitude and special appreciation to:

Carolyn DRAKE who revised the manuscript, Bertille DEJOUANY, Nathalie LOUIS, Nathalie PICAN for their outstanding assistance, and Monique DUCHATEAU and Sylvie DOYON, ANPEA, for their efficiency in organizing the meeting.

List of authors
Liste des auteurs

Barker Philip, Interactive Systems Research Group, School of Information Engineering, University of Teesside, Middlesbrough, Cleveland TS1 3BA, United Kingdom, phone : 44 (642) 34 26 60, fax : 44 (642) 23 05 27

Berliss Jane, Berkeley Systems, 2095 Rose street, Berkeley, CA 94709, USA, phone : 1 (510) 540 55 35, fax : 1 (510) 540 51 15

Béroule Dominique, LIMSI-CNRS, Université de Paris Sud, BP 133, 91403 Orsay cedex, France, phone : 33 (1) 69 85 80 64, fax : 33 (1) 69 85 80 88

Burger Dominique, INSERM U 88, groupe CREARE, 91, boulevard de l'Hôpital, 75634 Paris cedex 13, France, phone 33 (1) 40 65 98 99, fax : 33 (1) 45 83 83 02

Burnod Yves, INSERM groupe CREARE, Institut des Neurosciences, 9, quai Saint-Bernard, 75252 Paris cedex 05, France, phone 33 (1) 44 27 37 47, fax : 33 (1) 44 07 15 85

Cesarano Serge, CNEFEI, 58-60, avenue des Landes, 92150 Suresnes, France, phone 33 (1) 42 04 39 62, fax : 33 (1) 45 06 39 93

Denis Michel, LIMSI-CNRS, Université de Paris Sud, BP 133, 91403 Orsay cedex, France, phone : 33 (1) 69 85 80 08, fax : 33 (1) 69 85 80 88

Edwards Alistair, Department of Computing Sciences, University of York, York YO1 5DD, United Kingdom, phone : 44 (904) 43 27 22, fax : 44 (904) 43 27 67

Fluhr Christian, INSTN-GITD, bât. 528, CEN Saclay, 91191 Gif/Yvette, France, phone : 33 (1) 69 08 70 93, fax : 33 (1) 69 08 26 69

Hatwell Yvette, Laboratoire de Psychologie Expérimentale, Université de Grenoble II, BP 47X, 38040 Grenoble cedex, France, phone : 33 (76) 82 56 74, fax : 33 (76) 82 56 65

Hinton Ron, Tactile Diagram Research Unit, Education Department, Loughborough University of Technology, Loughborough LE11 3TU, United Kingdom, phone : 44 (509) 22 27 70, fax : 44 (509) 23 19 48

Martin Jean-Claude, LIMSI-CNRS, Université de Paris Sud, BP 133, 91403 Orsay cedex, France, phone 33 (1) 69 85 81 04, fax : 33 (1) 69 85 80 88

Mazurier Christian, CNEFEI, 58-60, avenue des Landes, 92150 Suresnes, France, phone : 33 (1) 42 04 39 62, fax : 33 (1) 45 06 39 93

Roby-Brami Agnès, INSERM, groupe CREARE, Institut des Neurosciences, 9, quai Saint-Bernard, 75252 Paris cedex 05, France, phone : 33 (1) 44 27 34 40, fax : 33 (1) 44 07 15 85

Sagot Jacques, CNEFEI, 58-60, avenue des Landes, 92150 Suresnes, France, phone : 33 (1) 42 04 39 62, fax : 33 (1) 45 06 39 93

Sperandio Jean-Claude, Université René-Descartes, 28, rue Serpente, 75006 Paris, France, phone : 33 (1) 40 51 98 13, fax : 33 (1) 40 51 70 85

Stevens Robert, Department of Computing Sciences, University of York, York YO1 5DD, United Kingdom, phone : 44 (904) 43 27 22, fax : 44 (904) 43 27 67

Contents
Sommaire

V   Foreword
VII   Préface
XI   List of authors
     Liste des auteurs

    I. PERCEPTION, LANGUAGE AND REPRESENTATIONS
    I. PERCEPTION, LANGAGE ET REPRÉSENTATIONS

3   **Michel Denis**
    Visual images as models of described environments
    Les images visuelles comme modèles d'environnement décrits

13 **Yvette Hatwell**
    Images and non-visual spatial representations in the blind
    Images et représentations non visuelles de l'espace chez l'aveugle

37 **Yves Burnod**
    Scene analysis and linguistic description: from images to words
    Analyse de scènes et description linguistique : des images aux mots

    II. THE ILLUSION OF MANIPULABLE OBJECTS
    II. L'ILLUSION D'OBJETS MANIPULABLES

55 **Philip G. Barker**
    Pictorial communication
    Communication pictographique

79 **Agnès Roby-Brami**
    Direct manipulation of data
    Manipulation directe des données

97 **Dominique Burger, Christian Mazurier, Serge Cesarano, Jack Sagot**
The design of interactive auditory learning tools
Conception d'environnements sonores interactifs pour l'enseignement

III. CONSTRUCTION OF NEW INTERFACES
III. NOUVEAUX PRINCIPES DANS LA CONSTRUCTION D'INTERFACES

117 **Jean-Claude Sperandio**
Prospects for objects and standards in the interaction between computers and blind users
Perspectives pour le développement d'objets et de standards d'interfaces accessibles aux personnes aveugles

131 **Jane Berliss**
Software solutions to the problem of GUI inaccessibility to blind persons
Solutions logicielles au problème de l'inaccessibilité des interfaces graphiques pour les personnes aveugles

145 **Jean-Claude Martin, Dominique Béroule**
Trends in human-computer multi-modal interaction
Tendances actuelles dans le développement des interfaces multi-modales

IV. ACCESS TO TEXTS AND IMAGES
IV. ACCÈS AUX TEXTES ET AUX IMAGES

169 **Ronald A.L. Hinton**
Tactile and audio-tactile images as vehicles for learning
Images tactiles et audio-tactiles comme support d'enseignement

181 **Alistair D.N. Edwards, Robert D. Stevens**
Mathematical representations: graphs, curves and formulas
Représentations mathématiques : graphiques, courbes et formules

195 **Christian Fluhr**
Methods of text presentation
Méthodes de présentation des textes

Perception, Language and Representations

*Alice had never been in a court of justice,
but she had read about them in books,
and she was quite pleased to find
that she knew the name fo nearly
everthing there.
"That's a judge", she said to herself,
"because of his great wig."*

Lewis Carroll

Visual images a models of described environments

Michel Denis

Equipe Cognition Humaine, LIMSI-CNRS, Université de Paris-Sud, BP 133, 91403 Orsay Cedex, France

ABSTRACT

This paper reports some of the empirical efforts developed over the past twenty years by cognitive psychologists to assess the functional and structural properties of visual images, as well as their similarities to visual perception. The paper focuses more specifically on the processes involved in the construction of visual images from verbal descriptions, and provides a summary of findings supporting the claim that the processing of verbal information can generate mental representations similar to those constructed from visual perception.

Although the mind's capacity to reconstruct the visual appearances of the outer world has been a preoccupation since ancient times, modern science has only really been looking into mental imagery for the last twenty years with the ambition to produce claims validated by systematic empirical observation. Elaborating scientific knowledge about entities which are not accessible to direct observation is a particularly difficult challenge, and one which holds true for all internal mechanisms and representations that cognitive psychology attempts to account for. In the field of imagery, a long tradition mainly based on introspection was followed by the behaviorist dismissal of "mental chimeras", which has now been supplanted by approaches aimed at c aracterizing the cognitive processes governing the generation and manipulation of imaginal representations (see Denis, 1991 ; Kosslyn, 1983 ; Logie & Denis, 1991 ; Paivio, 1991 ; Shepard & Cooper, 1982). Most contemporary models of cognitive architecture include components purported to account for the mind's capacity to process visual images, in addition to other modality-specific representations as well as linguistic or more abstract forms of representation (e.g., Anderson, 1990 ; Baddeley, 1990).

THE EMPIRICAL INVESTIGATION OF MENTAL IMAGERY

The main paradigms used in imagery research adhere to the premise that scientific knowledge about internal events relies exclusively on adequately selected behavioral measures. Note that these paradigms all employ the same general technique where a subject is required to form a visual mental image, and the experimenter records a specific aspect of the subject's behavior. The scientist builds inferences from observed behavioral regularities about the (inner) mechanisms that are assumed to occur when such behavior is observed.

There are three major categories of imagery experiments. The first covers studies which record physiological measures in subjects who are currently forming or inspecting mental images of objects or visual scenes. A number of such measures have been investigated, such as electrodermal response, heart rate, eye movements, pupillary dilation. The idea underlying these approaches is that even though images cannot be accessed by external observation, these measures may provide objective counterparts of the internal processes behind image generation. These experiments tend to show that electrodermal response and heart rate are influenced by the content of images (especially their emotional content), that eye movements accompany the generation of images of moving objects, and so on. Although most of these indicators elicited a great deal of curiosity and enthusiasm on the part of researchers in early modern imagery research, they do not shed much light on the image itself and its intrinsic characteristics. Furthermore, these indicators may reflect other aspects than the image proper. For instance, variations in pupillary dilation are also found when subjects are engaged in non-imaginal tasks (such as mental calculation). Rather, they reflect the cognitive difficulty associated with the task being processed.

Studies which attempt to capture brain activity which accompanies the formation of mental images come closer in exploring the inner mechanisms governing imagery. For instance, it has been shown that there is a decrease of the alpha rythm in the occipital region when subjects produce visual images. There is converging evidence from studies based on the recording of evoked potentials, which also indicate that cerebral regions involved in the processing of visual information are also activated when subjects generate visual images. More recently, measures of blood flow variations confirm the role of the associative regions of the visual cortex in the generation of visual images (e.g., Charlot, Tzourio, Zilbovicius, Mazoyer & Denis, 1992 ; Goldenberg, Artner & Podreka, 1991).

Another kind of approach to the understanding of images is to investigate their potential effects on psychological activities, such as verbal comprehension, memorization, reasoning, or problem solving. The typical approach, here, consists in comparing two situations. In the control condition, subjects are simply required to solve a problem or perform a task. In the experimental condition, subjects are presented with the same task, with additional instructions to create as vivid images as possible of the data to be processed while performing the task. Comparing the output of the two conditions serves to respond to a very simple question: Do subjects perform better (that is, more rapidly or with fewer errors) when they use imagery than in the control condition ?

A number of empirical studies have shown that imagery indeed affects the processing of information in a positive way, at least when this information is likely to be expressed in the form of visual images.

For instance, memory for lists of concrete words benefits considerably from visualization of the objects referred to by these words. Memory for narratives is enhanced when readers are instructed to elaborate visual images of the characters, scenes, and actions described. In a variant on this paradigm, only one condition is examined : the condition without any imagery instructions. The comparison is made between those subjects who can be qualified as "high imagers" (based on adequate psychometric instruments, such as imagery questionnaires or visuo-spatial tests) and "poor imagers". In most cognitive tasks, people who exhibit a strong spontaneous tendency to visual imagery perform better than poor imagers.

The fact that imagery produces effects on cognitive processing, as is shown by these studies, leads directly to the issue of understanding the origins of these effects. What are the intrinsic properties which confer functional properties on images ? Probably one of the strongest cognitive enhancing effects of visual imagery is to facilitate the processing of objects that are not available to direct perception. This, by the way, is true of mental representations in general, inasmuch as they extend people's capacities of dealing with objects at a distance. This effect, however, is only manifest when a sufficient degree of isomorphism is achieved between the represented object and the representation, which makes it possible to perform valid computations on the latter. The analog property of imagery is probably its most valuable feature.

The third approach to imagery does not investigate this process either for its physiological counterparts or for its effects on cognitive functioning, but for its own putative structural properties. The functional approach is complemented here by a structural approach, which consists in producing claims about the properties and internal structure of imaginal experiences. The most illustrative experiments in this respect are those which evidence the "spatial" character of images, that is, their capacity to preserve the metric properties of the objects they stand for. The main paradigms are those based on mental scanning or mental comparison. Another related line of research consists in analyzing the temporal characteristics of imagery. Chronometric analyses here inform us on the processes by which images are generated, the processes governing their maintenance, and those responsible for their transformations (such as mental rotation). These lines of research are generally developed within more comprehensive and articulated models of cognitive architecture, and they now tend to rely heavily on the investigation of the brain structures responsible for these processes (cf. Farah, 1988 ; Kosslyn, 1988 ; Tippett, 1992). A dominant research trend consists in assessing the functional and structural similarities between imagery and perception. The next section reports now classic, well-established findings from a few selected experiments intended to assess such similarities, as well as functional interactions between imagery and perception.

FUNCTIONAL AND STRUCTURAL SIMILARITIES BETWEEN IMAGERY AND PERCEPTION

Imagery and perception share several features, if only at the phenomenal level, in that both make a certain kind of visual experience available to the individual. Objective measures, in addition, are collected in order to assess the similarities, and possibly the commonalities, of the processing mechanisms recruited in both cases.

A straightforward paradigm, here, consists in comparing two conditions. In the first condition, the subject is invited to perform a given task and is placed in direct contact with the object or configuration on which this task is based. In the second condition, the subject has to perform the same task, with the instruction to visualize this object or configuration, which means that at the time the task is performed, the only available information is an internally generated image. If the perceptual condition has any effects, will the imaginal condition produce any effects as well ? If so, will the effects in the imaginal condition occur in the same direction and with the same magnitude as in the perceptual condition ?

One example is found in a study on the memorization of imagined or visually presented objects (Denis, 1975). It has long been established that the memorization of a list of concrete words, either presented in a written form or auditorily, is enhanced when these words are accompanied by drawings or photographs of the objects designated by these words. The new condition examined here consisted in presenting subjects with a list of nouns to memorize, with the additional instruction to form mental images of the corresponding objects. The results show that not only memorization with imagery produces positive effects on recall, just as is the case in picture memorization, but also that these effects are of similar magnitude in both conditions. Thus, perceptually processed information and internally generated information appear to have similar effects in terms of mnemonic encoding.

A major finding was reported by Margaret Peterson (1975). In her study, the experimenter presented subjects with a 4 x 4 matrix, of which 12 cells were filled by an uppercase letter of the alphabet. After subjects had studied this material, the matrix was withdrawn from their sight and they were invited to reconstruct it from memory on an empty matrix. A finding of special interest here was that the proportion of correct recall varied to a great extent as a function of the cell position in the matrix. Cells located at the periphery were better recalled than those in the center of the matrix, and more particularly the four corner cells. This hierarchy of recall probability was replicated in full in a condition where subjects only saw the empty matrix and were instructed to imagine which letter was in which cell (upon listening to verbal assignment of letters to specified cells).

A further relevant example can be found in a set of experiments designed by Podgorny and Shepard (1978) to compare pattern-analyzing mechanisms involved when a subject either imagines a visual configuration or is presented with this configuration perceptually. In the perceptual condition, the subject was shown a grid of 5 x 5 cells on which a block letter was displayed, resulting from the darkening of several cells. Immediately after the block letter was removed, a colored dot appeared on one of the cells of the grid. The subject had to decide whether this dot appeared on a cell which was occupied by the letter or a formerly empty cell. Podgorny and Shepard recorded subjects' response times. Analysis of these times revealed several regularities. In particular, response times varied as a function of the structural complexity of the letter (e.g., "E" vs. "I"). They also varied as a function of the part of the letter where the dot was located. Furthermore, when the dot appeared on a cell which had not been darkened, response times varied as a function of the distance between this cell and the cells occupied by the letter. To summarize, the speed of responses (as well as their accuracy) was highly dependent on structural variables of the figural pattern which had been perceived.

Podgorny and Shepard extended this task to an imaginary condition. In this condition, subjects did not see any letter appearing on the grid, but they were instructed to mentally "darken" the appropriate cells in response to the auditory presentation of a given letter. Then the colored dot appeared, and the subjects were to decide whether the dot occupied one of the cells on which the letter was visualized. The analysis of responses reveals the very same chronometric regularities as in the perceptual condition, depending on the very same structural variables. Response times only tended to be longer in the imaginal condition, but the overall pattern of results was otherwise identical. These findings clearly suggest that similar pattern-analyzing mechanisms are implemented in the visual system when subjects observe an object and when they imagine the same object (even though the degree of activation of these mechanisms is presumably higher in the perceptual condition).

The last example comes from experiments which compared perceptual vs. mental scanning of visuo-spatial configurations (cf. Denis & Cocude, 1989). In the perceptual condition, subjects were presented the map of an island which showed several geographical features on its periphery (a harbor, a lighthouse, a creek, a hut, a beach, a cave). Subjects were invited to visually focus on one specific feature (for instance, the harbor). When hearing the name of another feature (for instance, the beach), the subjects were required to perform visual scanning in a straight line to this feature, and to depress a button when they reached it. Not surprisingly, the results show a linear relationship between scanning times and the distances separating features.

In another condition, another group of subjects were instructed to learn the map to a point where they were capable of drawing it from memory accurately. Subjects were then invited to form a visual image of the map and to perform purely mental scanning. Results show that scanning times exhibited the same linear relationship with distances as in the perceptual condition. This finding indicates that when information on a bidimensional object is represented in the form of a visual image, the internal organization of this representation preserves the spatial structure of the original object, and in particular the relative distances among its parts (provided sufficient learning has been devoted to the construction of the image). Thus, imagery may provide people with cognitive events which can be used in a way similar to perceptual events, and elicit cognitive responses that closely resemble those produced in perceptual situations. Images not only contain information, but at least in some respects, the manipulation of this information is quite similar to the manipulation of visual percepts.

Lastly, if images and percepts involve similar mechanisms, their interactions should have predictable effects when both are implemented at the same time, in the direction of either facilitation (when the figural contents of both experiences are compatible) or interference (when figural contents are different). For instance, in an experiment reported by Martha Farah (1985), subjects were invited to form the visual image of a capital letter, for instance "H". Simultaneously to this imagery task, subjects were asked to perform a visual detection of faintly presented letters. In some cases, the letter to be detected was the same as the letter currently imagined by the subject (in this example, "H"). In other cases, it was a different letter (for instance, "T"). The results show that subjects are more likely to visually detect a letter which is the same as the letter they are imagining at the same time. This finding reinforces the assumption that common representational structures are activated during imagery and perceptual processing.

THE VISUALIZATION OF OBJECTS FROM VERBAL DESCRIPTIONS

In the perspective reported above, imagery is considered to be a surrogate process by which the mind self-generates internal experiences that more or less reproduce or reconstruct previous perceptual experiences. This "reproductive" and in some extreme cases quasi-photographic type of imagery does not however exhaust the scope of the functions of imagery. Images also fulfill anticipatory functions, for instance when they are constructed by a subject who is expecting a forthcoming perceptual event. Imagery also has a creative function when it is involved in the process of inventing new objects or configurations, or in scientific discovery (cf. Shepard, 1988).

Besides images constructed from perception, imagery may also be involved in situations devoid of any particular visual input. A number of our daily imaginal experiences occur in situations where we receive verbal descriptions of objects, persons, scenes or events, without any perceptual contact with them. Nevertheless, we are able to construct at least approximate, and in some cases rather accurate, representations which despite their non-perceptual origin, are experienced as having visual content. These representations, in addition, can be used to plan and execute appropriate actions, as is the case when we construct cognitive maps of unknown environments described by another person and follow routes in these environments. Obviously, the quality of the representation and consequently its usefulness largely depend on the speakers' capacities to produce adequately structured discourse.

Although there is no doubt that people are able to construct visual images of non-perceived, solely described objects, the question remains whether such representations possess characteristics which make them really similar to perceptually based images or whether they must be considered as specific sorts of visual images. In order to answer this question, the experiment reported above on the mental scanning of imagined configurations was extended to a condition where subjects were initially presented with a short text describing the island to be memorized. The description told about a map of an island which was circular in shape, with several geographical features located on the periphery. Locations were unambiguously defined in the conventional hour-dial terms of flight navigation ("At 11 o'clock, there is a harbor. At 1, there is a lighthouse. (...)"). One group of subjects heard the description three times. Another group of subjects heard the same description six times. After having listened to the description, the subjects were asked to perform mental scanning according to the same instructions as before.

Subjects in both groups produced scanning times which revealed a significant positive relationship between scanning times and imagined distances. However, subjects who heard the description three times exhibited a lower time-distance relationship than those who processed the text six times, but these latter subjects produced responses which did not differ from those of subjects who learned the map perceptually. In addition, after three learning trials, scanning times tended to be longer than those of subjects who learned the map from perceptual inspection, but this difference disappeared after three more learning trials. Although the verbal information could be recalled accurately after three trials, the spatial qualities of the visual image at this time appeared to be imperfectly consolidated, resulting in a rather low time-distance correlation. These results suggest that images constructed from verbal descriptions progress toward a stable, high-resolution state, the equivalent of the state attained more rapidly by images derived from perception.

In a subsequent series of experiments (Denis & Cocude, 1992), the effects of the structure of the description were investigated. One group of subjects were presented with a well-structured text. Geographical details were introduced in a highly predictable, consistent sequence, namely, in clockwise order. Another group listened to a version of the description which was designed to make it difficult for subjects to incorporate details in the outline structure of the island. In this version, sentences were presented in a random sequence. Such a sequence was expected to create more demanding conditions during the formation of an image (although not basically impeding its elaboration), and presumably would take longer to reach the end state of a stable, well-defined image than would well-structured descriptions.

The results replicate the time-distance relationship when the image was constructed from the well-structured description, but not when the image was generated from three repetitions of the random description. Six exposures to the randomly ordered information yielded the expected time-distance relationship in image scanning. A likely interpretation is that additional exposure to the poorly structured information allowed the image to develop the structural coherence and resolution needed to support consistent scanning. Thus, the structure of descriptions can affect the intrinsic structure of images of described objects and hence the mental operations performed subsequently on these images.

Mental scanning is just one of the many sorts of mental operations that a person can be required to perform on visual images with chronometric outputs likely to reflect the isomorphism of these images to the objects they represent. Another task of interest is the mental comparison of distances separating the main points of the configuration. For instance, is the distance between the harbor and the beach longer or shorter than the distance between the harbor and the cave ? Such comparisons of visually presented stimuli are known to produce a "symbolic distance effect" ; that is, the larger the difference between two distances, the shorter the time needed to respond. This effect holds when subjects perform size comparisons of familiar objects from memory. For instance, is a horse bigger than a zebra ?

In one further experiment (Denis & Zimmer, 1992), subjects performed mental comparisons of distances after having either studied the map of the island or listened to its verbal description. The results show that subjects in both conditions presented equally high levels of performance. Furthermore, a clear effect of the magnitude of the difference was found for both groups of subjects, with performance steadily increasing from comparisons involving small differences to those involving large differences. Subjects who learned the description of the island also showed response times which decreased linearly with increased difference between compared distances. This effect provides grounds for the claim that representations constructed by subjects from verbal descriptions possess intrinsic properties that are isomorphic to those of physical spatial configurations. In addition, it is worth mentioning that subjects with the highest imagery capacities are those who apparently benefit the most from situations where images are to be constructed from discourse. High visuo-spatial imagers are overall more accurate than low imagers in distance comparisons, and their response times are overall significantly shorter.

This indicates that people with strong tendencies towards visualization can convert verbal descriptions into vivid images wherein information is accurately displayed and easily accessed.

Thus, verbal information effectively allows people to construct representations which entertain structural isomorphism with described objects, as do images resulting from perceptual processing of these objects. Equally important, the representation constructed from text or discourse not only contains those pieces of information which were explicitly stated (for instance, that there is a harbor at a given location), but also contains metric information which was not made explicit at any time in the text or discourse (information regarding the relative distances between features). The capacity of description-based images to display non-explicit information derives from an important representational property inherent in visual imagery ; that is, specifying locations of subparts of the representation necessarily makes the relative positions of these subparts evident.

There are a number of situations where people can take advantage of their imagery capacities to construct visual representations of spatial configurations from discourse. This is the case in particular when people have to construct visual representations of two-dimensional patterns, such as chess positions (cf. Saariluoma, 1989), or to create mental models of three-dimensional spatial environments (cf. Franklin, Tversky, & Coon, 1992 ; Taylor & Tversky, 1992).

FURTHER RESEARCH DIRECTIONS

A number of fields remain underexplored in the domain of imagery. Within the issues described in this paper, a promising line of research would be to further investigate the processes by which people create mental models of unseen environments from text or discourse. Language is an especially flexible tool which allows people to externalize their internal representations in order to have other people share these representations. Language also enables people to transmit configurations that are unavailable to other people's perception for some reason (for instance, the configuration is simply unavailable, or there is considerable distance between the configuration and the observer, or the observer's processing system is not functional, either temporarily or permanently). In particular, more active research should be developed to understand how blind people construct representations of their environments, in particular through linguistic communication (cf. Carreiras & Codina, 1992 ; Cornoldi, De Beni, Roncari, & Romano, 1989).

Another line of research which is obviously complementary to research on the comprehension of verbal descriptions consists in investigating the processes involved in the generation of these descriptions. Language is inherently sequential, which entails that in the description of complex objects, speakers have to choose the order in which the different parts of these objects will be entered into their discourse. This makes it particularly relevant to analyze the various strategies that can be used in descriptions, and to identify whether some of them are "better" than others in terms of communicative efficiency. It is also important to define the cognitive factors which constrain the selection of some descriptive strategies (cf. Robin & Denis, 1991). This should help identify the cognitive characteristics of naturally proficient describers, and to propose devices to improve speakers' and writers' descriptive abilities.

REFERENCES

Anderson J. R. (1990), *The adaptive character of thought*, Hillsdale, NJ: Lawrence Erlbaum Associates.

Baddeley A. (1990), *Human memory : Theory and practice*, Hillsdale, NJ: Lawrence Erlbaum Associates.

Carreiras, M. & Codina B. (1992), Spatial cognition of the blind and sighted: visual and amodal hypotheses, *European Bulletin of Cognitive Psychology, 12*, p.51-78.

Charlot V., Tzourio N., Zilbovicius M., Mazoyer B. & Denis M. (1992), Different mental imagery abilities result in different regional cerebral blood flow activation patterns during cognitive tasks, *Neuropsychologia, 30*, p.565-580.

Cornoldi C., De Beni R., Roncari S. & Romano S. (1989), The effects of imagery instructions on total congenital blind recall, *European Journal of Cognitive Psychology, 1*, p.321-331.

Denis M. (1975), *Représentation imagée et activité de mémorisation*, Paris : Editions du CNRS.

Denis M. (1991), *Image and cognition*, New York : Harvester Wheatsheaf.

Denis M. & Cocude M. (1989), Scanning visual images generated from verbal descriptions, *European Journal of Cognitive Psychology, 1*, p.293-307.

Denis M. & Cocude M. (1992), Structural properties of visual images constructed from poorly or well-structured verbal descriptions, *Memory and Cognition, 20*, p.497-506.

Denis M. & Zimmer H. D. (1992), Analog properties of cognitive maps constructed from verbal descriptions, *Psychological Research, 54*, p.286-298.

Farah M. J. (1985), Psychophysical evidence for a shared representational medium for mental images and percepts, *Journal of Experimental Psychology : General, 114*, p.91-103.

Farah M. J. (1988), Is visual imagery really visual? Overlooked evidence from neuropsychology, *Psychological Review, 95*, p.307-317.

Franklin N., Tversky B. & Coon V. (1992), Switching points of view in spatial mental models, *Memory and Cognition, 20*, p.507-518.

Goldenberg G., Artner C. & Podreka I. (1991), Image generation and the territory of the left posterior cerebral artery, In R. H. Logie & M. Denis (Eds.), *Mental images in human cognition* , Amsterdam : North-Holland, p.383-395.

Kosslyn S. M. (1983), *Ghosts in the mind's machine : Creating and using images in the brain*, New York : W. W. Norton.

Kosslyn S. M. (1988), Aspects of a cognitive neuroscience of mental imagery, *Science, 240*, p.1621-1626.

Logie R. H. & Denis M. (Eds.) (1991), *Mental images in human cognition*. Amsterdam : North-Holland.

Paivio A. (1991), *Images in mind : The evolution of a theory*, New York : Harvester Wheatsheaf.

Peterson M. J. (1975), The retention of imagined and seen spatial matrices, *Cognitive Psychology, 7,* p.181-193.

Podgorny P. & Shepard R. N. (1978), Functional representations common to visual perception and imagination, *Journal of Experimental Psychology : Human Perception and Performance, 4,* p.21-35.

Robin F. & Denis M. (1991), Description of perceived or imagined spatial networks, In R. H. Logie & M. Denis (Eds.), *Mental images in human cognition* , Amsterdam : North-Holland, p. 141-152.

Saariluoma P. (1989), Chess players' recall of auditorily presented chess positions, *European Journal of Cognitive Psychology, 1,* p.309-320.

Shepard R. N. (1988), The imagination of the scientist, In K. Egan & D. Nadaner (Eds.), *Imagination and education* , New York : Teachers College Press, p. 153-185.

Shepard R. N. & Cooper L. A. (1982), *Mental images and their transformations*. Cambridge, MA : The MIT Press.

Taylor H. A. & Tversky B. (1992), Spatial mental models derived from survey and route descriptions, *Journal of Memory and Language, 31,* p.261-292.

Tippett L. J. (1992), The generation of visual images : A review of neuropsychological research and theory, *Psychological Bulletin, 112,* p.415-432.

Résumé

L'article présente un bilan succinct des travaux expérimentaux menés au cours des vingt dernières années en psychologie cognitive en vue de mettre en évidence les propriétés fonctionnelles et structurales des images mentales visuelles, ainsi que leur similitude avec la perception. Une attention particulière est accordée aux processus mis en oeuvre dans la construction d'images visuelles à partir de descriptions verbales. Les résultats des expériences rapportées fournissent des arguments en faveur de l'hypothèse selon laquelle le traitement de l'information verbale permet de générer des représentations mentales similaires à celles dérivées de la perception.

Images and non-visual spatial representations in the blind

Yvette Hatwell

Laboratoire de Psychologie Expérimentale, Université Pierre-Mendès-France, BP 47, 38040 Grenoble Cedex 9, France

ABSTRACT

According to Kosslyn (1980, 1990), mental images are a specific form of internal representation and their cognitive processes are similar to those involved in perception. In order to study images and more generally non-visual representations in the blind, it is therefore necessary to know how total congenital blindness affects perceptual processes and knowledge. In the first section, the perceptual development of sighted and blind infants, children and adults is studied with special emphasis on the interactions between vision, audition and haptics. It was shown that the visual-haptic cross-modal integration at work very early in infancy gives the blindfolded sighted an advantage over the congenitally blind in spatial perceptions and representations. A similar lasting advantage was manifest in the late blind whose blindness occurred after the age of 3-4 years.

The second section concerns imagery in the blind. Research has revealed that congenitally blind people can generate and use mental (non-visual) images in the same way as the sighted, but that the blind suffer from imagery limitations due to their spatial perceptual deficit and to the high attentional load associated with processing of imaged spatial data. Similarly, studies showed that congenitally blind children can recognise simple tactual raised line drawings and that texts illustrated with tactile pictures were recalled better than unillustrated texts. However, when the processing of these tactile pictures captured too much attention in the blind, it impaired semantic processing. In conclusion, these observations are discussed in relation to educational practices and to the use of graphic devices by the blind.

INTRODUCTION

Studies on the effects of total congenital blindness on the cognitive development of children and adults have focused over the last few decades on spatial perceptions and representations, since early visual deprivation mainly impairs sensorimotor and conceptual spatial functioning. More recently, processes underlying this spatial deficit have been investigated in relation to the problem of the imaged versus propositional format of mental representations in the blind. Do congenitally blind people form and manipulate mental images in the same way as sighted people manipulate visual images? If so, what is the psychological status of these non-visual mental images and to what extent can these images help in the elaboration of technical devices providing cognitive aids for the blind?

In sighted people, mental images are predominantly visual, although spatial knowledge is also provided by other perceptual systems. Consequently, research on imagery has concentrated on visual images. Some authors (Pylyshyn, 1973, 1981) theorised that mental images are encoded in the same abstract propositional format as the one used to encode verbal information. Other researchers (Kosslyn, 1976, 1980) have argued that mental images are a specific form of internal representation and that their cognitive processes are similar to those involved in perception. Accordingly, Kosslyn (1990) defined visual imagery as "seeing in the absence of the appropriate sensory input" (p.73) and assumed that images are "perceptions of remembered information", with the restriction that the remembered information should have visual properties that cannot be inferred from other stored information. In this conception, visual imagery studies necessarily include comparisons between the processing of sensory inputs (perception) and the processing of the imagined corresponding data (mental images).

Studies of mental imagery in people completely blind from birth may provide some insights in this debate, since early blindness does not affect language acquisition and semantic processing, while it does result in important perceptual impairment. If mental imagery is closely linked to perception (mainly visual) as claimed by Kosslyn, then congenitally blind subjects should behave differently from sighted subjects in tasks implying imagery.

In order to study imagery in blind people, the cognitive consequences of early blindness must first be evaluated. Which perceptual systems are still available in blindness and to what extent do these systems provide the same knowledge as the visual system? The present paper will therefore be divided into two sections. In the first, the development of perception and representations is examined in the sighted and in the blind, with special emphasis on the interactions between the spatial perceptual systems, i.e. on cross-modal integration. Once the nature of the perceptual handicap resulting from blindness is evaluated, it will be possible to focus on imagery studies in the blind. Consequently, the second section of this paper will analyse recent work comparing the characteristics of mental imagery in congenitally and in late blind subjects.

DEVELOPMENT OF SPATIAL PERCEPTION AND REPRESENTATIONS

The perceptual systems in the sighted

a) Each of the perceptual systems available in human beings is specialised in the processing of some kind of information (Freides, 1974; Pick, 1974). Vision is the spatial sense *par excellence*: It has a wide perceptual field allowing the processing of simultaneous stimulation, its foveal discrimination abilities are very high and it provides a continuous flow of stimulation in its peripheric field which regulates posture and locomotion.

The proximo-receptors of the haptic (tactilo-kinesthetic) system are only activated when they are directly in contact with the stimulus. As a result, the haptic perceptual field is considerably reduced compared with the visual field and large exploratory hand movements are necessary in order to perceive objects in their entirety. This means that haptic perception is much more sequential than visual perception. Nevertheless, when stimulus size and location are adequate for manual exploration, haptics provide very similar kinds of spatial and physical information to vision (shape, size, localisation, orientation, texture, etc.). But as a spatial sense, haptics is less performant than vision even in adults (Hatwell, 1986; Klatzky & Lederman, 1987). It is mainly used in the sensori-motor loop regulating motor actions on the environment (Freides, 1974) and, according to Lederman et al. (1986), it is specialised in the perception of substance properties of objects (texture, hardness, etc).

Audition also provides spatial information, especially concerning the localisation and movements of sound sources, but in this domain it is consistently less performant than vision. Audition is functionally specialised in the processing of sequential (temporal) stimulation and its role is particularly crucial for accessing spoken language.

Finally, muscular and articular proprioception provide information about the position and movements of the body or segments of it. Its role is fundamental to motor control and it is also involved in haptic perception since exploratory movements are necessarily involved in haptics.

How do these perceptual systems function and evolve from birth? How do they cooordinate in order to provide unified knowledge about the external world? We will first consider infancy, followed by childhood and adulthood.

b) Recent studies on infant perception have revealed that the peripheral visual system is already functional at birth. In contrast, the focal system is much more immature, but matures rapidly during the first three months of life. As a result, vision in new-born infants is more performant than has been thought in the past. Very young infants discriminate two- and three-dimensional objects, they discriminate changes in location, slant, visual texture, etc. However, up to the age of 3-4 months, infants perceive figures as the addition of separate elements while by 4-5 months, they begin to organise these elements into structured configurations, as do older children and adults.

The haptic system evolves more slowly during infancy. Up to the age of two months, tactual perceptions are mainly oral because of the immaturity of the pyramidal motor pathways which precludes the voluntary control of arm and hand movements. By one month of age, young infants differentiate orally the texture and shape of nipples when they suck and explore them with their mouth (Meltzoff & Borton, 1979; Rochat, 1983). Concerning manual haptic perception, correct shape discrimination (a plain square versus a square with a hole in its centre) was observed at 2-3 months of age in infants prevented from seeing their hands exploring these objects (Streri, 1987). These haptic manual discriminations improve consistently during the first year of life, but they remain generally less performant than the corresponding visual perceptions (for a review, see Streri, 1991).

As concerns cross-modal co-ordination between the spatial perceptual systems, recent studies have revealed that, contrary to what was assumed in the past (Piaget, 1936), sensory spaces are not independent in infancy. They interact and communicate from birth, although intermodal relations are different in the new-born and in older infants, children and adults.

For example, a rough and rigid visual-manual co-ordination functions at birth, was first observed by Bower (Bower, 1974) and then evidenced with more methodological controls by von Hofsten (1982, 1984). This author showed that when a visual target is presented to new-born babies, they extend their arm in the direction of the target but do not reach and contact it. This arm extension elicited by a visual stimulus implies cross-modal transfer between the eyes and the hands, since the visual perception of the target location has to be communicated to the arm in order to program its movement in the correct spatial direction. This early "pre-reaching" behaviour (von Hofsten, 1984) disappears by 6-7 weeks of age and reappears at approximately 5 months with new characteristics. At this age, the rate of contact with the target is high and reaching movements are controlled by sensory reafferences (visual and proprioceptive). From 5-6 month onwards, hand actions are systematically guided and controlled by vision, and the perceptual (haptic) function of the hand becomes definitely subordinated to its motor instrumental function (for a review, see Hatwell, 1986; Streri, 1991).

Cross-modal transfer of shape discrimination between haptics and vision and between vision and haptics was first demonstrated by Gottfried, Rose and Bridger (1977) and Rose, Gottfried and Bridger (1981) in 12-month-old infants. More recent studies showed that this transfer occurs earlier. Streri (1987) habituated 2-3 month-old infants to a shape presented haptically in one of their hands and then she presented visually either the familiar shape or a novel shape. The infants fixated visually longer the novel shape, showing that their haptic familiarity with the old shape was transferred to vision. However, cross-modal transfer in the reverse direction, i.e. from vision to touch, was observed only by 5-6 months of age.

Similarly, vision and audition communicate at birth. Muir & Field (1979) and Wertheimer (1961) observed that new-born babies rotated their head and eyes in the direction of a non-visible toy sounding laterally. This means that information concerning the auditory target location was transferred to other perceptual systems.

According to Bower (1974) and to Humphrey et al. (1988), this early auditory-visual co-ordination disappears by 6-8 weeks and reappears at approximately 4-5 months.

Cross-modal co-ordination between audition and prehension is more difficult to achieve than cross-modal co-ordination implying vision. Bower (1974) and Stack et al (1989) observed that uptil 9-10 months of age, infants placed in a dark room do not extend their arm in the direction of a sounding toy in order to grasp it (remember that the co-ordination of vision and prehension is achieved at 5 months). This developmental lag between vision and audition demonstrates the superiority of vision in space perception. The co-ordination of the two less performant spatial systems (ears and hands) is consistently delayed compared to the co-ordination of vision with one of these less performant spatial modalities.

However, these studies demonstrated that visual and non-visual perceptions are integrated from birth onwards and that the knowledge gathered by one perceptual modality may be transferred very early to other modalities. Consequently, the spatial abilities of the haptic and auditory systems in the sighted are systematically enriched by visual knowledge transferred to them through vision.

c) In children and adults, consistent improvements are observed in intramodal discrimination abilities of each of the perceptual modalities described above, and at these ages the functional specialisation of these modalities is always more apparent than in infancy. The dominance of vision over the other modalities in spatial perception is evidenced in a number of experimental situations, the most obvious being what happens when two modalities are in conflict. For example, Rock & Victor (1964) asked adults to palpate a square shape under a curtain while they simultaneously saw this object through a lens reducing the horizontal dimension of the square. Consequently, the block appeared visually as a rectangle and haptically as a square. When asked to recognise the shape of the block they had seen and touched simultaneously, the subjects systematically choose the rectangle which corresponded exactly to the visual one. This means that haptic perception was ignored or recalibrated on the visual input ("visual capture"). The same results were observed in 5 year-old children (McGurk & Power, 1980) and even in adult potters whose professional job had highly developed their haptic perceptions (Power & Graham, 1976). Similarly, visual capture is often observed in vision-proprioception and in vision-audition conflicts involving spatial localisation of a target.

In contrast, if the task concerns temporal perceptions (rhythmic structures, for example) or if it is verbal and implies linguistic material, audition dominates vision and perceptual conflicts are solved by auditory capture (Freides, 1974). The domain in which haptics is dominant is less salient. However, Lederman, Klatzky and Reed (1987) observed a tendency towards haptic capture in a texture discrimination task in which vision and haptics were in conflict. This means that when substance perception is concerned, haptic perceptions are valued more than visual ones, while the reverse is true in spatial perception.

This suggests that data conveyed by the non-dominant system are recoded in the code of the dominant modality and are adjusted to it. Since vision is dominant in spatial perception, non-visual spatial information (haptic and auditory) tends to be coded visually. In contrast, sequential data and particularly linguistic material are recoded in the auditory code if they are perceived visually (Freides, 1974; Hatwell, 1986 and in press (a); Pick, 1974).

The development of spatial perception and representations in the blind

What happens when complete blindness occurs at birth? How do people deprived early of one of the most important perceptual systems adapt to the physical environment and access spatial knowledge?

Audition and haptics are the main sources of perception in the blind. As already stated, both convey spatial information and could therefore compensate for visual deprivation, at least partly. However, the crucial role of audition in blindness is to allow language learning and therefore to give access to higher conceptual thinking and to social communication. As for haptics, it is the best substitute for vision, although it cannot reach the same level of spatial performance as vision. Let us now examine the development of spatial knowledge, first in congenitally blind infants and then in older children and adults.

a) Generally speaking, the sensorimotor development of blind infants does not differ from the development of sighted infants except in regards to spatial behaviour.

During the first two or three months of life, totally blind babies do not markedly differ from sighted ones. By 3 months of age, a progressive and persistent general hypotonia appears in blind infants (Bullinger & Mellier, 1988), which results from the absence of the continuous peripheral flow of stimulation provided by vision. Contrary to what would be expected, blind infants do not spontaneously manifest an intense manual exploratory activity; their hands are often retracted at shoulder level with they finger in the air, or they are pushed in their eyes ("blindisms"). Only systematic haptic stimulation provided by the mother will lead blind infants to use their hands as perceptual organs able to gather knowledge about the environment.

Spatial impairment is first manifest in prehensile behaviour. Fraiberg's (Fraiberg et al, 1966; Fraiberg, 1977) and Bigelow's (1986) observations on the development of the co-ordination of audition and prehension in blind infants showed that this co-ordination occurred at the end of the first year of life, i.e. at the same moment as in normally sighted babies. But sighted babies take considerable advantage of vision-manual co-ordination much earlier, as was described above. Since blind babies are deprived of this spatial experience, there is a developmental lag of approximately 5 months in the emergence of directed reaching in blind infants compared with sighted ones.

Autonomous locomotion is another behaviour seriously affected by early blindness. Blind babies walk without aid at about 20 months (Fraiberg, 1977) and some children may walk alone only by 25-30 months, although they do not suffer from any motor, neurological or mental defects (Bigelow, 1986). The deprivation of the continuous flow of stimulation provided by vision, which regulates posture and cinetic equilibrium and facilitates anticipation of obstacles and planning of the locomotor path, is difficult to compensate by auditory and haptic cues in blind infants.

Some technical aids, like the UltraSonic Guide (Kay, 1974), tend to overcome these limitations by substituting the lacking continuous visual flow by a corresponding continuous auditory flow. Many studies have shown that the use of this "sonar" by blind infants consistently helped them, although this help only occurred during certain periods in their development (Sampaio, 1989; Bullinger & Mellier, 1988).

On the other hand, blindness has no effect on language development and blind babies do not differ from sighted ones in this domain. As soon as they access this major symbolic instrument, blind children develop this mode of communication and they often tend to advantage verbal knowledge over perceptual knowledge ("verbalism") since, for them, the latter is more effortful than the former.

Finally, it is noteworthy that in partial blindness or in amblyopia, i.e. in infants who benefit from some residual visual acuity, spatial impairment is consistently less important than in total blindness. This demonstrates once again the role of vision as a spatial perceptual system.

b) In pre-school and school-aged children, spatial impairments are observed at the perceptual and representational levels. Haptic spatial perceptions of congenitally blind children are systematically less efficient than the corresponding visual perceptions of the sighted, and they are also less efficient than haptic spatial perceptions of blindfolded sighted children. This is observed in shape, size, localisation, distance and orientation discriminations (for a review, Hatwell, 1978, 1986 and in press b). Thus, although the congenitally blind are highly pratised in the use of the haptic perceptual system, they are nevertheless impaired in relation to the blindfolded sighted who rarely use haptics without seeing. It is likely that this impairment stems from the lack of visual representations which are transferred to haptics when sighted people are temporarily deprived of vision.

This assumption is supported by the fact that late blind children and adults (i.e. people whose complete blindness occurred after the age of 3-4 years of age) do not manifest the same handicap in spatial perceptions as the congenitally blind. For them, haptic discriminations do not differ from those of blindfolded sighted subjects, although in some cases the late blind have no conscious memory of visual images because of their early loss of vision. This means that visual-haptic cross-modal transfer that took place during infancy definitely modified the haptic perceptual system and this gain is maintained throughout life even if total blindness occurs later.

Two examples will illustrate the nature of the difficulties encountered by congenitally blind children and adults in spatial perception and representations. Both concern the spatial consequences of a movement on target localisation.

The first example is taken from Rieser's work. Rieser (1990) reported a study conducted by Talor, Garing and Rieser in which six congenitally blind children, aged 2 to 5 years, were placed in the centre of a circle. Eight identical boxes were positioned on its circumference at equidistant locations. After a familiarisation phase in which the child explored the apparatus with the experimenter, a toy was given to the child and was placed by the child (with the aid of the experimenter) in one of the boxes. Afterwhich the child was taken back to the centre of the circle and his/her body was oriented exactly in front of the target box containing the toy. Then, the child was gently rotated by either 90° or 270° and the experimenter asked him/her to face the target box.

If a spatial map of the apparatus has been constructed, the child will perform the shortest possible movement bringing him/her in front of the target. When the initial body rotation was 90°, this shortest movement was a 90° movement in the reverse direction. But when the body rotation was 270°, the shortest movement was a 90° movement prolonging the initial rotation in the same direction (Fig. 1).

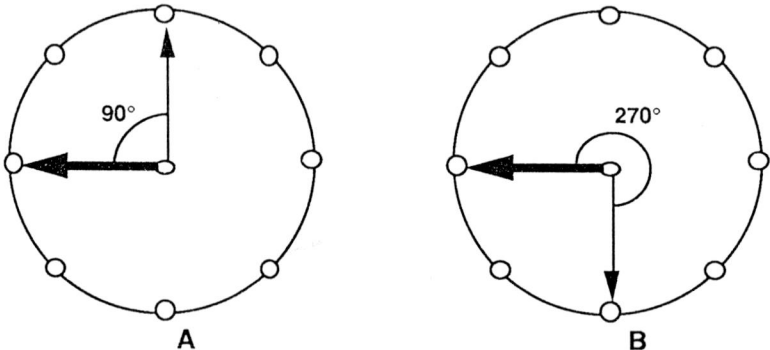

Fig. 1. *The experimental situations tested by Rieser. A) the child is rotated 90°. B) the child is rotated 270° (Adapted from Rieser, 1990).*

Only one congenitally blind child showed this economic spatial strategy and he/she was the oldest, aged 5 years. The five other children turned back in front of the target by performing a 270° rotation in the reverse direction of the initial rotation, showing therefore that they had not constructed a useful cognitive map of the environment.

The same task was presented to sighted children aged 25 months. After a visual presentation of the apparatus, the room was darkened and the children were tested in the same conditions as the blind. In the 270° rotation condition, all of them returned in front of the target box by rotating 90° in the same direction as the initial rotation.

This showed that, while sighted children processed both the movements achieved and the spatial consequences of these movements, blind children seemed to process only the movements and did not take into account their spatial effects.

The second example concerns adults. Lederman, Klatzky and Barber (1985) studied in early and late blind subjects the estimation of the euclidian distance between two points (i.e. the shortest distance between them) when, with the index of one hand, the subject moved from one point to the other along a detour path. The length of this sinuous (Fig. 2) path was a multiple (either 4 or 8 times) of the euclidian distance to be estimated. If the movement actually achieved from the starting point to the end point is coded instead of the euclidian distance between these points (this euclidian distance was never directly explored haptically), then the estimated euclidian distance would vary as a function of the length of the detour path. Results supported this prediction both in early and in late blind adults. But, as shown in Fig. 3, this effect was greater in congenitally blind subjects. Once again, early visual-haptic cross-modal integration that took place in the late blind during the first years of their life gave them a permanent advantage over the early blind.

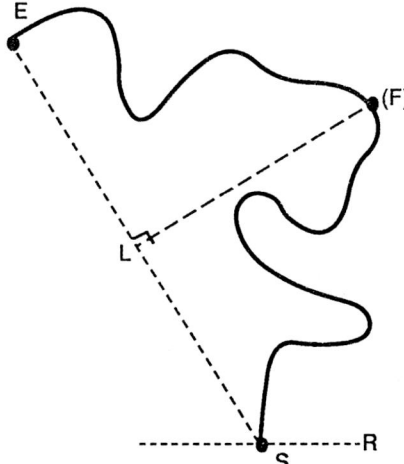

Fig. 2. The detour path achieved by the index finger of the subject, and the euclidian distance (between points S and E) to be evaluated (Adapted from Lederman, Klatzky and Barber, 1985).

In sighted subjects performing a similar task in the visual modality (in this condition, a small light was running along the detour path in a darkened room), an overestimation of the euclidian distance as a function of the length of the detour path was still observed, but its magnitude was consistently smaller than in the blind (Balakrishnan, Klatzky, Loomis & Lederman, 1989). This shows that the general modes of coding are similar in vision and in haptics but that in haptics, the tendency to rely on movement coding is significantly greater than in vision. As a result, the spatial consequences of movements are often not taken into account in congenitally blind people.

In conclusion, the main cognitive consequences of blindness concern spatial perception and representations, and these spatial difficulties are markedly more important in early blind than in late blind. However, although they suffer from this developmental lag, it is noteworthy that congenitally blind people achieve spatial concepts and spatial behaviour that are not fundamentally different from those of sighted people. This means that blindness affects the speed of development of spatial behaviour and the strategies of spatial coding, but not the very content of spatial knowledge.

We can now return to the question raised in the introduction: do congenitally blind people rely on images closely related to their perceptions, as do the sighted according to Kosslyn (1973, 1990)?

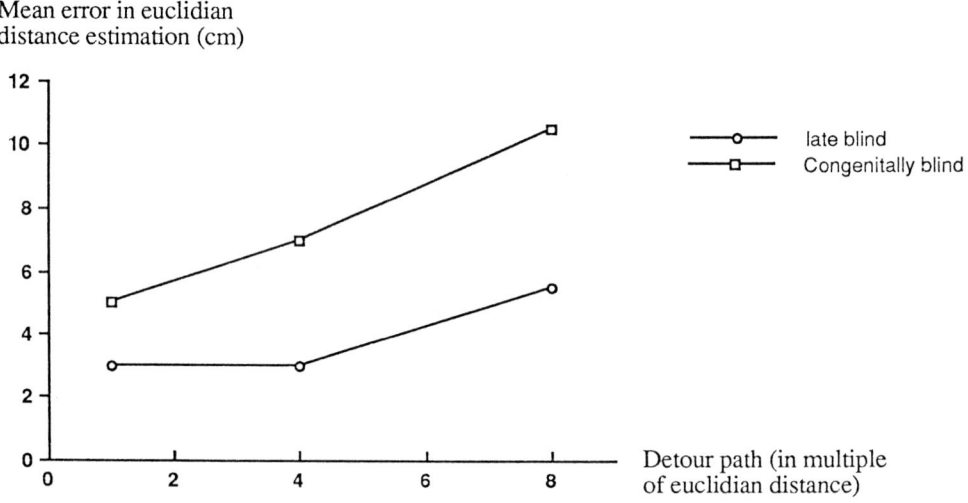

Fig.3. Mean errors in the estimation of euclidian distance as a function of the length of the detour path (in multiples of euclidian distance) in congenital and in late blind adults. (Adapted from Lederman, Klatzky & Barber, 1985).

IMAGES AND THE BLIND

Studies on mental imagery will be considered first and then we will describe research showing how blind people use pictorial images which represent, in a bi-dimensional format, the tri-dimensional objects of our world.

Mental imagery in the blind

a) The earlier direction of research on mental imagery in the blind concerned the role of imagery instructions on the verbal memory of paired associate words.

In this task, a list of paired words are presented and subjects are asked to recall the word associated with each target word. Paivio (1969, 1971) claimed that concrete words were easier to remember than abstract words because they aroused images that facilitate the associative processing necessary for good memory performance. Although more often visual, these images could also take on other modalities if the referent of the word was primarily perceived in another modality ("modality-specific imagery" hypothesis). For example, *rainbow* would evoke visual images while *thunder* would evoke auditory images.

Paivio & Okavita (1971) assumed that since the congenitally blind lack visual images, they should find the concrete words whose referents are purely visual to be as difficult to recall as abstract words. Consequently, these subjects should perform more poorly than sighted subjects on the concrete words for which they cannot create images. Results showed that, as assumed by the authors, the blind recalled fewer high-visual- than high-auditory-imagery pairs, whereas the reverse occurred in the sighted. However, in contrast with the predictions, there was no difference between the blind and the sighted in the number of high-visual pairs recalled. In further studies (Hans, 1974; Kerr, 1983; Zimmler & Keenan, 1983), the results of Paivio & Okavita were not replicated: The blind performed better in high-visual- than in high-auditory-imagery words, and there was no difference between groups in the recall of words referring to things that could be seen but not touched (i.e. *rainbow*). Similarly, Jonides et al. (1975) observed that when presented with paired-associate lists composed of high-imagery concrete words versus low-imagery abstract words, instructions to use imagery resulted in the same facilitation of recall in blind and in sighted subjects. Furthermore, the amount of facilitation was the same for the concrete and the abstract words. These results were interpreted as showing that both the sighted and the blind used semantic representations, and that in both groups instructions to image were treated as instructions to elaborate these semantic representations.

The conclusions of this set of studies were questioned more recently by DeBeni & Cornoldi (1988) because, according to these authors, all of them rely on the following incorrect reasoning: When the observed performances of the congenitally blind are the same as those of the sighted, or when blind subjects do not perform as predicted by the assumed imagery content of the words, this means that visual imagery was not implied in these tasks. The fallacy of this argument stems from the fact that what was labelled "visual images" by the experimenters did not result necessarily and exclusively from visual perception. Instead, these so-called visual images could be based on information collected through different perceptual modalities. The visual object properties are mixed with other spatial, textural or configural properties not derived from vision. Consequently, the problem should not be whether congenitally blind people use images of visual objets such as a *rainbow* (obviously, they do so through the non-visual components of these images), but what are the limitations of imagery in early blind subjects as compared to sighted ones. If Kosslyn was correct in assuming that mental images have the same characteristics as the corresponding perceptions, then the blind should perform poorer than the sighted in imagery tasks that rely mainly on their handicapped perceptual domain.

DeBeni & Cornoldi (1988) therefore presented congenitally blind and sighted adults with a task in which a locative word (*bathroom, street,* etc) was associated either with another single word, or with a pair of words, or with a triplet of words. The list was composed of high-imagery concrete nouns or of low-imagery abstract nouns. The task was to recall the word(s) associated with the target. In order to improve memory performance, subjects were instructed to form interactive images linking the words of each single, pair or triplet item. Results showed that in both groups high-imagery words were recalled better than low-imagery words and that, for the single condition, the blind performed as well as the sighted. Differences between the two populations appeared however in the triplet condition: while in the sighted the number of words recalled in the correct order improved in this condition as compared to the pair condition, performance decreased in the blind when the number of words associated with the target increased (Fig. 4). In contrast, the blind and sighted did not differ when order of recall was not taken into account, i.e. when correct responses were given in a scattered way. These results suggested that congenitally blind people accessed imagery and used it in a similar way to the sighted, but that they had consistent limitations in this domain when interactive images and memory for order were implied.

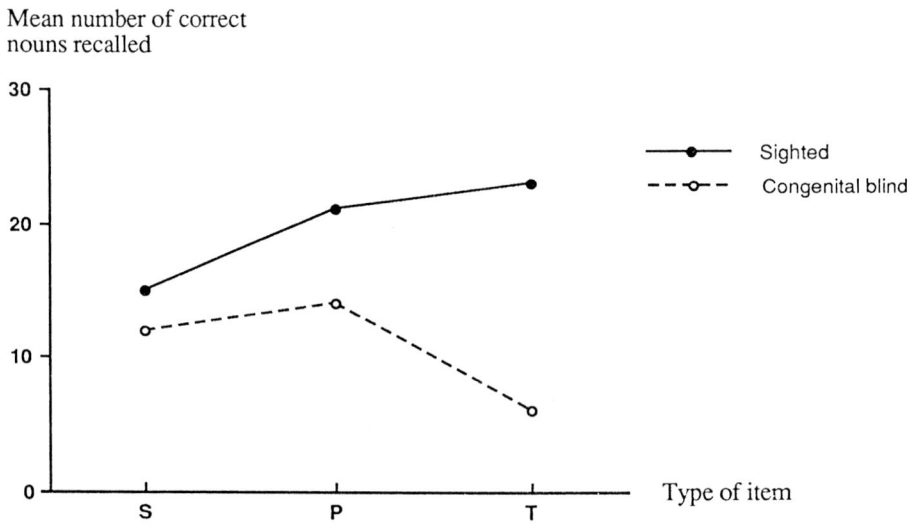

Fig.4. Mean number of nouns recalled (in order) when presented in singles, pairs or triplets by congenitally blind and late blind adults. S = singles, P = pairs, T = triplets (Adapted from DeBeni & Cornoldi, 1988).

b) In another direction of research, imagery was more directly studied in non-verbal tasks of the kind proposed by Cooper & Shepard (1973) to sighted subjects. These authors presented adults with a drawing of a complex tri-dimensional geometric figure coupled with another figure which was either the same as the original but in another orientation, or was a mirror image.

Subjects pressed one button if they judged that the comparison figure was the same as the standard and another if the comparison figure was a mirror. Results showed that when the two figures were the same, response time (RT) improved linearly as a function of the orientation of the comparison. This means that subjects mentally rotated the latter until it matched the standard figure, and this mental rotation of visual images took more time when the magnitude of slant of the comparison figure increased.

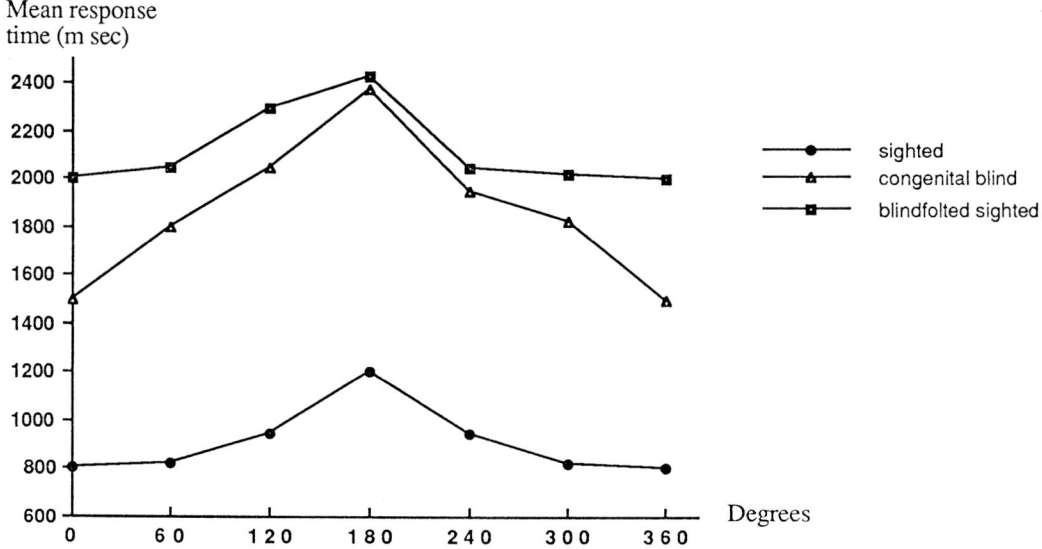

Fig. 5. *Mean response time (in milliseconds) as a function of degree of rotation in congenitally blind, late blind and blindfolded sighted adults (Adapted from Carpenter and Eisenberg, 1978).*

Marmor & Zaback (1976) adapted this experimental paradigm to haptics and asked whether similar results are observed in congenitally blind, in late blind and in blindfolded sighted. A linear increase of RTs was observed in the three groups, but these RTs were higher in the congenitally blind than in the late blind. Similar observations were reported by Carpenter & Eisenberg (1978) (Fig. 5). The authors therefore concluded that mental rotation did not rely exclusively on visual images, and that the non-visual imagery at work in congenitally blind subjects had the same functional properties as the visually dominant imagery of the sighted, but that imagined rotations were slower in the blind than in the sighted.

c) Imagery in the blind has also been studied in tasks implying the processing of bi- or tri-dimensional spatial information of imagined objects, and loading more or less working memory. Adapting Kerr's (1987) task and procedure, Cornoldi et al. (1991) asked congenitally blind and sighted adults to imagine a matrice composed of bi-dimensional squares or of tri-dimensional cubes. These matrices could be either 3 x 3, 4 x 4 or 8 x 8 (if bi-dimensional), or 2 x 2 x 2, 3 x 3 x 3 or 4 x 4 x 4 (if tri-dimensional).

One element of the matrix was taken as the starting point (for example the cube near the right side of the subject). The subject had to follow the path of this element mentally while the experimenter described its movement ("two steps left, one step upward", etc.), and to point to its final position. When the matrices were bi-dimensional, the blind performed as well as the sighted. In the tri-dimensional matrices of low and medium complexity (2 x 2 x 2 and 3 x 3 x 3), there were more errors in the blind than in the sighted. But in the most complex matrice (4 x 4 x 4), performances were equally poor in both groups (Fig. 6).

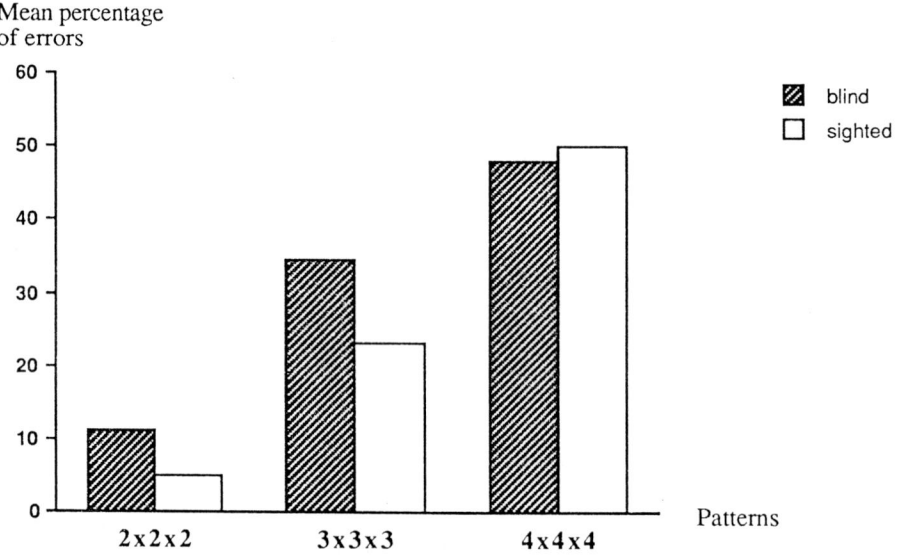

Fig.6. Mean percentages of errors on three-dimensional patterns in congenitally blind and sighted adults (adapted from Cornoldi et al., 1991)

This demonstrated that sighted subjects took advantage of their high level abilities in imagery processes, but that these processes were involved mainly in the easier tasks. When the spatial complexity of the matrix was too high, both groups switched to other modes of coding, probably based on semantic and propositional processing.

In order to test the assumption that visual imagery did not help the processing of the more complex matrix, another group of sighted adults was presented with the same task but, in addition, a visual interfering stimulation (an intermittent light turned on randomly) was provided while the subject mentally followed the path of the element inside the matrix. The reasoning was that, if visual imagery was implied in this task, performances would be impaired by the visual interfering stimulation. Results confirmed this prediction, but only for the low (2 x 2 x 2) and medium (3 x 3 x 3) complexity matrices. In the more complex tri-dimensional matrix (4 x 4 x 4), there was no difference between the condition with the visual interfering task and the control condition without interference.

This confirmed that sighted people did not use visual imagery in a specific and exclusive way. When spatial patterns are too complex to be processed through imagery, other modes of coding may be elicited, especially abstract and semantic.

These observations demonstrated that congenitally blind people may generate spatial mental images and that in many cases, these images are not functionally different from those of the sighted. However, imagery limitations in the blind are demonstrated when task complexity increases.

d) Finally, in order to distinguish between the *spatial* (which may be non-visual) and the visual content of images, Arditi et al. (1988) presented tasks relying on a highly visual aspect of space perception, the property of perspective. Objects sustend different visual angles when seen at different distances, and this is known only through vision. Congenitally blind and sighted adults were therefore asked to form images of objects varying in size in the real world (an aspirin pill, a coffee cup, a motorcycle, a bus, etc). Subjects first estimated the apparent "distance" of these objects from them in any units they felt comfortable with. Secondly, they were asked to image the object at great distance and then to "move" towards it until (if at any time) it "overflowed" the image. Results showed that in both groups, large objects were imagined farther away than small objects, but this effect was consistently greater in the sighted than in the blind. The blind estimated the imaged objects to be significantly nearer to them than did the sighted. This observation suggested that since imagery in the blind is mainly mediated by haptics, it is restricted to the space of prehension. Finally, only one congenitally blind subject reported "overflowing" of the image, showing the specifically visual characteristic of overflowing.

In another experiment, Arditi et al. (1988) asked congenitally blind and sighted adults to point to the left (or the right) side of an object imaged at three distances from them (3, 10 and 30 feet). Visually, objects located far away sustend smaller visual angles than objects located near the subject. If this kind of perspective information is based on purely visual properties, the congenitally blind should not respond accurately in this task. Results confirmed this prediction. In both groups, pointing varied according to the size of the imagined objects. But pointing in sighted subjects also varied according to distance, while it did not in the blind.

Once more, this set of observations suggested that imagery in the blind has some aspects in common with imagery in the sighted, but that it differs from it on the purely visual components of visual images, such as perspective transformations.

Tactile pictures and the blind

In the preceding sections, we showed that congenitally blind people were generally delayed in the development of their spatial perceptions and that, correlatively, their imagery processes suffered from some limitations compared with those at work in sighted people. The last problem to be studied is whether raised tactile pictures are recognised by the blind as representing real objects and whether such tactile pictures may help them acquire knowledge about their environment.

Pictures are mainly visual representations since they are perspective bi-dimensional projections of tri-dimensional objects. Blind people have no sensory access to perspective transformations and, as reported earlier, their imagery does not take this visual property into account. Moreover, until recently, devices allowing the formation of raised pictures were scarce and consequently, blind people had a very restricted experience with raised drawings. However, Kennedy (1983) reported that congenitally blind subjects could recognise and produce tactile graphic pictures in which some pictural features, such as occluding boundaries, were processed correctly.

a) Some researchers have attempted to replicate these observations in order to know how the blind use tactile pictures. Pathak & Pring (1989) studied the ability to haptically recognise a target raised line picture among three comparisons in 13 year-old children. The subjects were not informed that the stimuli were in fact pictures of objects. These pictures represented only one face of a common object (i.e. there was no perspective transformation). In each trial, one of the distractors shared perceptual feature similarities with the target and the other distractor was random. For example, when the target picture was a *drum*, the featural distractor was a *tin* and the random one was an *ice lolly*. In half of the trials, the depicted objects could have been previously experienced through touch, while in the other half they could not be experienced in their totality through tactual exploration alone (*mountain, moon*, etc.). Results showed that although accuracy was high in both groups, the congenitally blind performed better than the blindfolded sighted and that in both groups, the featural distractor was chosen more often than the random one when an error was made. However, neither the blind nor the sighted noticed that the stimuli depicted common objects. Moreover, there was no difference in the blind between the experienced and non experienced objects. Consequently, this task seemed to have been processed only at a perceptual level.

Another group of children (same age) was further tested on a similar task, except that recognition of the target picture was now verbal instead of haptic. After the presentation of the haptic target picture, the subject was asked to select the word depicting the target among three words presented orally. Would this semantic information help the child to identify and memorise the pictures? Results revealed no difference between the congenitally blind and the sighted, nor between the experienced and the non experienced objects. However, as compared with the preceding experiment, the performances of the blind decreased when the haptic picture was to be matched to a word depicting it.

Finally, in a third experimental condition, the task was to memorise three haptic pictures (constructed in the same way as in the preceding conditions) and then to match one of these memorised pictures with a word presented orally by the experimenter. In this task, the blind performed worse than the sighted. However, there was again no difference between the experienced and non experienced objects.

This set of observations showed that the blind were able to extract and store tactual information provided by the two-dimensional drawings, but that their performances decreased when the semantic content and the memory load of the task increased.

While the blind were better than the sighted in the first perceptual recognition task, they performed as well as the sighted in the second task where a picture was to be matched to one of three words, and they were surpassed by the sighted in the third task where three pictures were to be memorised in order to match one of them with a word. This increasing difficulty of the tasks may stem from the high attentional investment achieved by the blind when they process haptic spatial perceptions. As a consequence of this attentional load, the simultaneous semantic coding which is easily achieved in the sighted may be impaired in the blind.

In addition, Heller (1989) found that in tasks similar to those just described, there was a consistent advantage of late blind over congenitally blind adults. This showed once more that early visual-haptic co-ordination resulted in lasting improvements of haptic spatial perceptions and representations.

b) In spite of their limitations, congenitally blind people have a better recall of the content of texts presented orally to them when these texts are illustrated by tactual graphic pictures than when they are not. This was demonstrated by Pring & Rusted (1985) who presented orally a series of texts each containing seven facts to congenitally blind and late blind subjects, aged 14 years. Three of them were illustrated by thermoform pictures and four were non-pictorial facts. For example, a particular animal was said to have *"curly horns"* (pictorial fact) and to *"live in Africa"* (non-pictorial fact). After one text was presented twice, recall was tested either immediately or after a 15-minute delay filled with a Braille writing task. The illustrated texts were better recalled than non-illustrated ones presented to control subjects. This effect of illustration appeared both in congenitally and in late blind subjects when recall occurred without delay. In this condition however, improvement in the illustrated condition was greater in the late blind than in the congenitally blind. When recall was delayed, the illustrated condition was performed better than the non-illustrated condition only in late blind subjects, and this improvement concerned only pictorial facts, not non-pictorial ones. In the delayed test condition, recall was better for the congenitally blind in the pictorial information in the illustrated condition and the non-pictorial information in the non-illustrated condition.

This revealed that in congenitally blind people, pictorial information enhanced verbal memory, probably because haptic pictures focused attention on some aspects of the text that would otherwise be neglected. But since the processing of haptic pictures captured the subject's attention, the non-pictorial information was relatively neglected in the illustrated condition. In contrast, in the non-illustrated condition, priority was given to the processing of non-pictorial information.

CONCLUSION

In the preceding sections, we first described the developmental characteristics of the spatial perceptions and representations of the totally blind as compared to those of sighted subjects.

Experimental studies showed that although the spatial knowledge achieved by the congenitally blind was not fundamentally different from the spatial knowledge of the sighted, spatial discriminations and representations were systematically poorer when blindness occurred early in life. Such a developmental lag was not observed in late blind subjects and this revealed the importance of cross-modal integration taking place in sighted infants during infancy. The occurrence of early visual-haptic cross-modal transfer enhances the haptic system's abilities especially as concerns accuracy in discrimination, structural organisation of sensory inputs and memory for configurations. This finding has obvious educational implications: since the advantage taken from early visual knowledge and early visual-haptic co-ordination will be maintained throughout life, visually impaired children should be trained to use their residual vision and to co-ordinate it with haptics in order to transfer visual knowledge to haptics. If total blindness occurs later, its consequences on spatial perception and representation will be less than in the totally congenitally blind.

Imagery in the blind was studied in the second section. Since images are considered to be derived from perception and therefore to have the same properties, it was not surprising to find that early blind subjects could generate and use images in the same way as sighted subjects. This means that mental images are not necessarily visual, although in the sighted their visual component is highly dominant. However, significant imagery limitations were observed in the congenitally blind compared to sighted people, and it is likely that these limitations stem from the poorer perceptual haptic knowledge of the former. In tasks requiring complex interactive mental images and which load memory, imagery processing is impaired in the congenitally blind. This should be taken into account when designing technical devices intended to help the blind to communicate with people and computers.

The same observation may be derived from studies on raised picture drawings for the blind. These studies showed that congenitally blind children, aged 13 years, could recognise simple tactile drawings and that texts illustred with tactile pictures were recalled better than unillustrated texts. However, the perceptual processing of haptic pictures may capture the attentional resources of the blind to such a degree that, correlatively, it results in an impairment in semantic processing. This was mainly observed in the congenitally blind, while the late blind again showed a systematic advantage over the congenitally blind in picture recognition and production. Consequently, tactual graphic devices proposed to the congenitally blind should not overload the perceptual and memory processes of this population, in order to allow abstract and semantic processing of the task to take place.

REFERENCES

Arditi A., Holtzman J.D. & Kosslyn S.M. (1988), Mental imagery and sensory experience in congenital blindness, *Neuropsychologia*, 26, p.1-12.

Balakrishnan J.D., Klatzky R.L., Loomis J. & Lederman S.J. (1989), Length distorsion of temporally entended visual displays: Similarity to haptic spatial perception, *Perception & Psychophysics*, 46, p.387-394.

Bower T.G.R. (1974), *Development in infancy.*, San Francisco: Freeman.

Bullinger A. & Mellier D. (1988), Influence de la cécité congénitale sur les conduites sensorimotrices chez l'enfant, *CPC-European Bulletin of Cognitive Psychology*, 8, p.191-203.

Carpenter P.A. & Eisenberg P. (1978), Mental rotation and the frame of reference in blind and sighted individuals, *Perception & Psychophysics*, 23, p.117-124.

Cooper L.A. & Shepard R.N.(1973), The time required to prepare for a rotated stimulus, *Memory & Cognition*, 1, p.246-250.

Cornoldi C., Cortesi A. & Preti D. (1991), Individual differences in the capcity limitations of visuospatial short-term memory: research on sighted and totally congenitally blind people, *Memory & Cognition*, 19, p.459-468.

DeBeni R. & Cornoldi C. (1988), Imagery limitations in totally congenitally blind subjects, *Journal of Experimental Psychology, Learning,,Memory & Cognition*, 14, p.650-655.

Fraiberg S. (1977), *Insights from the Blind*, London: Souvenir Press.

Fraiberg S., Siegel B.L. & Gibson R. (1966), The role of sound in the search behaviour of a blind infant, *Psychoanalytical study of the Child*, 21, p.327-357.

Freides D. (1974), Human information processing and sensory modality: Cross-modal functions, information complexity, memory and deficit, *Psychological Bulletin*, 81, p.284-310.

Gottfried A.W., Rose S.A. & Bridger W.H. (1977), Cross-modal transfer in human infants, *Child Development*, 48, p.118-124.

Hans M. (1974), Imagery and modality in paired associate learning in the blind, *Bulletin of the Psychonomic Society*, 4, p.22-24.

Hatwell Y. (1978), Form perception and related issues in blind humans, In *Handbook of Sensory Physiology*, Vol. 8: *Perception*, eds. R. Held, H.W. Leibowitz & H.L. Teuber, New York: Springer Verlag, p.489-519.

Hatwell Y. (1986), *Toucher l'espace. La main et la perception tactile de l'espace*, Lille: Presses Universitaires de Lille,

Hatwell Y. (in press, a), Transferts intermodaux et integration intermodale, In *Traité de Psychologie Expérimentale*, eds. M. Richelle, J. Requin & M. Robert. Paris: Presses Universitaires de France.

Hatwell Y. (in press, b), Les incidences cognitives de la déficience visuelle précoce, In *Traité de Psychiatrie de l'Enfant et de l'Adolescent* (2nd revised edition), eds. R. Diatkine, S. Leibovici & M. Soulé, Paris: Presses Universitaires de France.

Heller M.A. (1989), Picture and pattern perception in the sighted and the blind: the advantage of the late blind, *Perception*, 18, p.379-389.

Hofsten C. von (1982), Eye-hand co-ordination in the new-born, *Developmental Psychology*, 18, p.450-461.

Hofsten C. von (1984), Developmental changes in the organisation of prereaching movements, *Developmental Psychology*, 20, p.378-388.

Humphrey G.K., Dodwell P.C., Muir D.W. & Humphrey D.E. (1988), Can blind infants and children use sonar sensory aids? *Canadian Journal of Psychology*, 42, p.94-119.

Jonides J., Kahn R. & Rozin P. (1975), Imagery instructions improve memory in blind subjects, *Bulletin of the Psychonomic Society*, 5, p.424-426.

Kay L. (1974), A sonar aid to enhance spatial perception of the blind: Engineering design and evaluation, *Radio & Electronic Engineer*, 44, p.605-627.

Kennedy J.M. (1983), Haptic pictures, In *Tactual perception: A sourcebook*, eds. W. Schiff & E. Foulke. Cambridge: Cambridge University Press, p. 305-333.

Kerr N.H. (1983), The role of vision in "visual imagery" experiments: Evidence from the congenitally blind, *Journal of Experimental Psychology, General*, 112, p.265-277.

Kerr N.H. (1987), Locational representation in imagery: the third dimention, *Memory & Cognition*, 15, p.521-530.

Klatzky R.L. & Lederman S.J. (1987), The intelligent hand, In The Psychology of learning and motivation, Vol. 21, New York: Academic Press, p.121-151.

Kosslyn S.M. (1976), Can imagery be distinguished from other forms on internal representation? Evidence from studies of information retrival time, *Memory and Cognition*, 4, p.291-297.

Kosslyn S.M. (1980), *Image and Mind*, Cambridge, Mass.: Harvard University Press.

Kosslyn S.M. (1990), Mental imagery, In *Visual cognition and action: an invitation to cognitive science*, Vol. 2, eds. D.N. Osherson, S.M. Kosslyn & J.M. Hollerbach, Cambridge, Mass: The MIT Press, p.73-97.

Lederman S.J., Klatzky R.L. & Barber P.O. (1985), Spatial and movement-based heuristics for encoding pattern information from touch, *Journal of Experimental Psychology, General*, 114, p.33-49.

Lederman S.J., Thorne G. & Jones B. (1986), Perception of texture by touch: Multidimensionality and intersensory integration, *Journal of Experimental Psychology: Human Perception and Performance*, 12, p.169-180.

Marmor G.S. & Zaback L.A. (1976), Mental rotation by the blind: Does mental rotation depend on visual imagery? *Journal of Experimental Psychology: Human Perception & Performance*, 2, p.515-521.

McGurk H. & Power R.P. (1980), Intermodal co-ordination in young children: vision and touch, *Developmental Psychology*, 16, p.179-180.

Meltzoff A.N. & Borton R.W. (1979), Intermodal matching by human neonates, *Nature*, 282, p.403-404.

Muir D.W. & Field J. (1979), New-born infants orient to sounds, *Child Development*, 50, p.431-436.

Pathak K. & Pring L. (1989), Tactual picture recognition in congenitally blind and sighted children, *Applied Cognitive Psychology*, 3, p.337-350.

Piaget J. (1936), *La Naissance de l'intelligence chez l'enfant*, Neuchatel: Delachaux & Niestlé.

Paivio A. (1973), *Imagery and verbal processes*, New York: Holt, Rinehart & Winston.

Paivio A. (1986), *Mental representations*, New York: Oxford University Press.

Paivio A. & Okavita H.W. (1971), Word imagery modalities and associative learning in blind and sighted subjects, *Journal of Verbal Learning and Verbal Behaviour*, 10, p.506-510.

Pick H.L. (1974), Visual coding of non-visual spatial information, In *Perception*, eds. R.B. McLeod & H.L. Pick , Ithaca: Cornell University Press, p.153-165.

Power R.P. & Graham A. (1976), Dominance of touch by vision: Generalisation of the hypothesis to a tactually experienced population, *Perception*, 5, p.161-166.

Pring L. & Rusted J. (1985), Pictures for the blind: An investigation of the influence of pictures on recall of text by blind children, *British Journal od Developmental Psychology*, 3, p.41-45.

Pylyshyn Z.W. (1973), What the mind's eye telle the mind's brain: a critique of mental imagery, *Psychological Bulletin*, 80, p.1-24.

Pylyshyn Z.W. (1981), The imagery debate :Analogue media versus tacite knowledge, *Psychological Review*, 87, p.16-45.

Rieser J.J. (1990), Development of perceptual control while walking without vision: the calibration of perception and action, In *Sensory-motor organisation and development in infancy and early childhood*, eds. H. Bloch & B.I. Bertental. Dordrecht, Holland: Kluver Academic Press (NATO Series)

Rochat P. (1983), Oral touch in young infants: Responses to variation of nipple characteristics in the first months of life, *International Journal of Behavioral Development*, 6, p.123-133.

Rock I. & Victor J. (1964), Vision and touch: an experimentally conflict induced between the two senses, *Science*, 143, p.594-596.

Rose S.A., Gottfried A.W. & Bridger W.H. (1981), Cross-modal transfer and information processing by the sense of touch in infancy, *Developmental Psychology*, 17, p.90-98.

Sampaio E. (1989), Is there a critical age for using the SonicGuide with blind infants? *Journal of Visual Impairment and Blindness*, 83, p.105-108.

Stack D.M., Muir D., Sheriff F. & Roman J. (1989), Development of infant reaching in the dark to luminous and "invisible sounds", *Perception*, 18, p.69-82.

Streri A. (1987), Tactile discrimination of shape and intermodal transfer in 2-to-3-month-old infants, *British Journal of Developmental Psychology*, 5, p.213-220.

Streri A. (1991), *Voir, atteindre, toucher. Les relations entre la vision et le toucher chez le bébé*, Paris: Presses Universitaires de France.

Zimler J. & Keenan J.M. (1983), Imagery in the congenitally blind: how visual are visual images? *Journal of Experimental Psychology, Learning, Memory and Cognition*, 9, p.269-282.

Wertheimer M. (1961), Psychomotor co-ordination in auditory-visual space at birth, *Science*, 134, 1692.

Résumé

Selon Kosslyn (1980, 1990), les images mentales sont une forme spécifique de représentation et relèvent de processus cognitifs semblables à ceux des perceptions correspondantes. Pour étudier l'imagerie non visuelle chez les aveugles, il faut donc savoir au préalable quels sont les effets de la cécité complète précoce sur la connaissance perceptive de l'environnement. Dans la première section, l'étude du développement perceptif des nourrissons, des enfants et des adultes voyants et aveugles congénitaux fait ressortir l'importance de la coordination intermodale entre la vision, l'audition et le toucher. Cette coordination, qui se manifeste dès les premiers mois de la vie, enrichit les perceptions tactilokinesthésiques des voyants et donne à ces derniers un avantage sur les aveugles de naissance en ce qui concerne les perceptions et représentations spatiales. Cet avantage se retrouve aussi de façon permanente chez les aveugles tardifs qui ont perdu la vue après l'âge de 3-4 ans.

La seconde section porte sur l'imagerie chez les aveugles. Les travaux montrent que les aveugles précoces ont des images mentales (non visuelles) dont la fonction et l'utilisation sont semblables à celles des voyants. Cependant, les aveugles connaissent certaines limitations dans ce domaine en raison de leur déficit perceptif spatial et du coût attentionnel élevé associé chez eux au traitement des données spatiales imagées. De même, d'autres recherches montrent que les aveugles congénitaux peuvent reconnaître tactilement des dessins en relief et que des textes "illustrés" de dessins en relief sont mieux retenus que des textes non illustrés. Mais, si le traitement perceptif de ces dessins mobilise trop fortement l'attention, le traitement sémantique de ces dessins peut en être affecté. En conclusion, les implications de ces observations sont discutées en relation avec les pratiques éducatives et avec les aides techniques qui, aujourd'hui, font appel à l'imagerie et au dessin en relief chez les aveugles.

Scene analysis and linguistic description: from images to words

Yves Burnod

INSERM, Groupe CREARE, Neurosciences et Modélisation, Institut des Neurosciences, Université Pierre-et-Marie-Curie, 9, quai Saint-Bernard, 75252 Paris Cedex 05, France

ABSTRACT

Visual information about the surrounding environment can be communicated by the means of language. Recent neurobiological findings provide new insights into neuronal processes in the brain which relate images and words. A considerable research effort in signal processing, machine vision, artificial intelligence and artificial neural nets has been devoted to developing systems which transform images (pixels from stereo cameras) into words which can provide useful information about the environment. With the progress of miniaturization in computer technology, this research can result in environment-sensing devices providing real time useful information to people with a visual impairment: for example obstacle detection and avoidance or guidance cues in order to plan a safe path.

Our brain acquires information about the environment through several sensory and motor channels, either by direct interaction, such as visual recognition, or by communication with other people through language. People who have poor or no vision can learn language through auditory, tactile, proprioceptive and motor channels. They can thus communicate with other people about the visual content of the environment. Progress in computer speed and electronic miniaturization has lead to the development of vision-to-language aids for visually impaired people which provide real time information derived from vision through language communication: to explore the surrounding environment, to follow a safe path, to locate and reach needed objects (Blash, 1989; Adjaoui, 1992).

Three complementary questions can be asked in order to improve our understanding of the relationship between images and language:

• *What are the important and useful factors in the relationship between images and language?*
• *How does the brain to relate images and language?*
• *How can an artificial system be designed which transforms images (pixels from stereo cameras) into words, and what are we already able to do?*

WHAT ARE THE IMPORTANT AND USEFUL FACTORS IN THE RELATIONSHIP BETWEEN IMAGES AND LANGUAGE ?

The world surrounding a person can be described as a *scene* with objects in specific locations, people moving, informative signals: a village with houses and stores, a street with vehicles and people walking about, a room with familiar and useful objects, a working place with machines, a computer screen with icons and symbols....

Our brain is able to analyse these scenes and describe them with words. This process is not a simple image-to-word transformation which could be defined as a pixel-to-symbol mathematical formula. Furthermore, a complete objective description of a scene with words is perhaps not possible and is surely not necessary. Rather, scene description should be viewed as the result of the interactions between three main components of our brain (see following section & Fig. 1) that must be taken into account by any artificial system (see last section & Fig. 2):

• *Image processing*: Scene description requires the extraction of information from 2D images of the real world with a set of *image processing algorithms*: for example, the extraction of depth information from 2D images, the distinction between flat and upright surfaces, object identification, etc... (Marr, 1979). In the brain, these algorithms are performed by neural networks distributed in several cortical areas. In artificial systems, some of these algorithms are mastered (Horn, 1988 & 1989) and can be hardwired for real time processing (for example movement detection) (Sandini, 1990), others are still a matter of intense research and currently represent a bottleneck for possible applications (for example object recognition).

• *Goals and needs*: the relationship between images and language is not at all automatic but is directed, at any given time, by the *specific goals* of the observer: walking safely, learning the location of all objects in a room, manipulating icons on a computer screen. In the brain, these goals correspond to basic *sensorimotor and cognitive programs*. The design of artificial aids for visually impaired people should focus on applications responding to their demands: these demands can be expressed in terms of goals and needs which generally correspond to the main sensorimotor and cognitive programs of the brain.

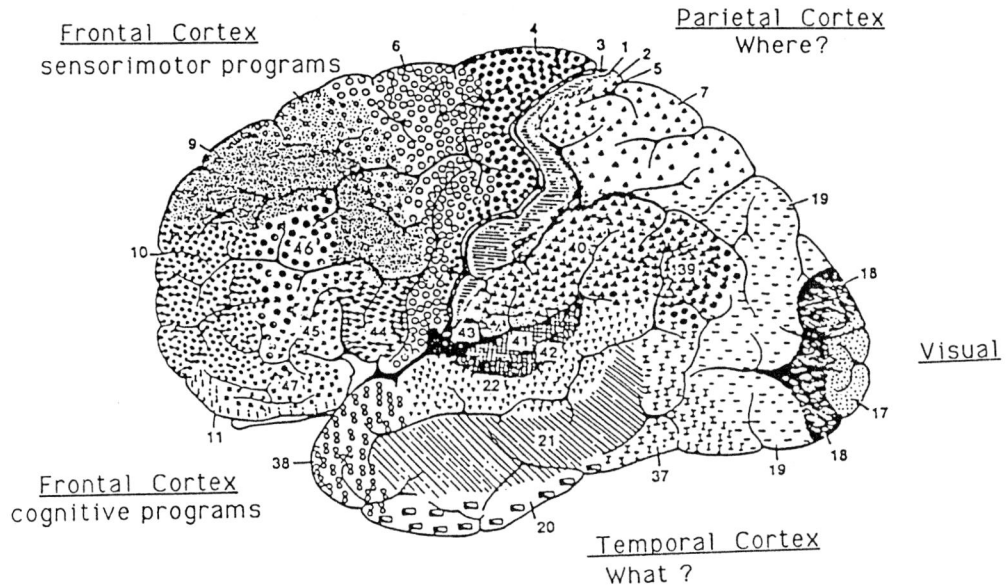
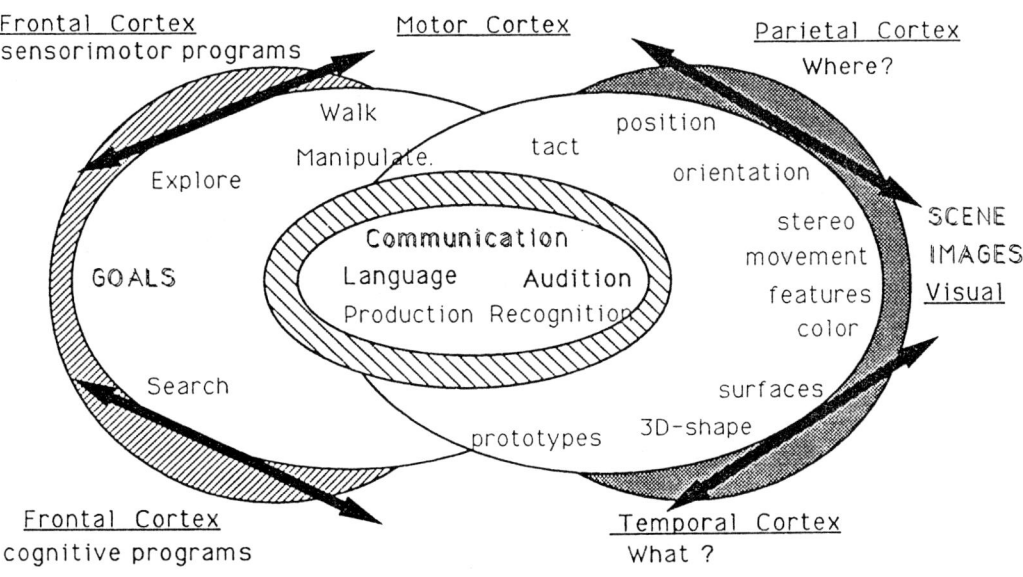

Figure 1

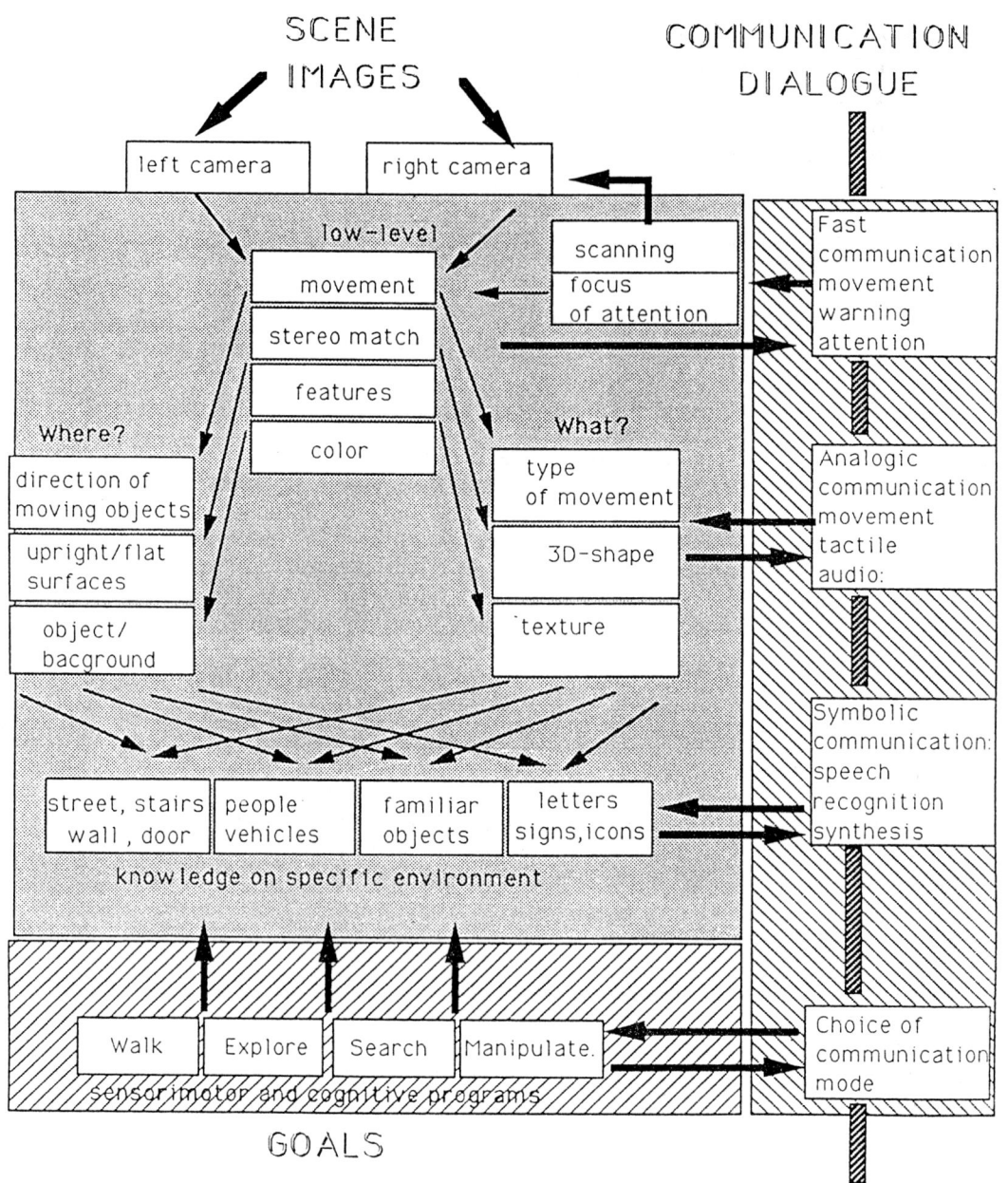

Figure 2

- *Communication*: Scene description is based on *a dialogue* with *questions* generated by the goals and needs, and *responses* generated by the results of the image processing algorithms in a given environment. In a single brain, such a dialogue naturally occurs between brain areas which represent goals (for example a sensorimotor programs such as walking or exploring), and brain areas which process visual information (Burnod, 1988). This *dialogue* is central for the design of artificial aids for visually impaired people: questions are asked by a person who can not see the direct relations with his goals and needs, and answers should be given by the artificial aid which has access to the visual content of the surrounding environment.

We have represented these three components of scene description (goals, visual processing and communication) in the same way both in the brain (Fig. 1) and in a artificial system (Fig. 2). It is hoped that this will answer basic goals and needs of visually impaired people.

The relationships between the specific needs of a person and the questions that can be answered from visual information are of great importance in scene description. For example, if my goal is to walk to a given place, several questions arise concerning what visual information can provide an answer: What is the best path? Are there any obstacles? If I am looking for a specific object, the question is: Where is this object? Is it in front of me? Some of the resulting questions can be directly answered by the outputs of image processing algorithms. Thus, this breakdown into questions allows scene analysis and provides a description with words.

Questions may be implicit and continually present: Is there a danger? Is there a new event? and in these cases the dialogue is initiated by a warning triggered when the response is positive. Implicit questions in the brain often correspond to the *emotional content* of a scene: movements can evoke fear, colours can provoke pleasure, people can generate desires, situations can provoke anger. These emotional contents cause direct reactions which completely modify the way a scene will be described: for example, if the meaning is "danger", the whole scene analysis is immediately directed to how to react to this danger. *Novelty* and event detection is a permanent process which can interrupt ongoing programs such as walking, talking or exploring.

Scene description is also constrained by subgoals, such as the duration of the description: one can describe the same scene with three words or ten books: at the one extreme, the presence of a danger may lead to an immediate and short warning ("be careful"!), and at the other extreme, a very long and precise exploration of a scene may be a pleasure in itself. Between these two extremes, time is proportional to the precision of the description necessary to answer a specific question.

Natural vision is never passive but always interactive. The direct projection of light on the retina depends on eye position and more generally upon the *point of view* that can be controlled actively at any time: by moving eyes in order to change the focus of attention; by manipulating, in order to isolate and analyse an object; by changing lighting conditions; by walking in order to change the distance. Artificial vision attempts to imitate these interactions and is becoming increasingly active.

In order to design visual aids, it is important to identify what is common to everyone, and what is specific to an individual. *Previous knowledge* (that which is stored in the brain) completely modifies the way we perceive our environment. As previous knowledge increases, information from the retina can be less and less precise, more and more noisy, and exploration can take less and less time. A great deal of knowledge is acquired during early childhood from sensori-motor interactions with the environment and depends on the sensori-motor channels used.

This knowledge allows the transformation of the pixel content of an image into a guide for motor action: Can I walk on this path? Is there a shadow or a textured background, or a vertical object which is an obstacle? These questions can be answered from the pixel content of the image, in a similar way for everybody. Such *a common experience* can also be integrated into algorithms of artificial systems, and has been, for example, widely used in the autonomous control of mobile robots.

To this common knowledge, each person adds *personal experience* depending on past history and everyday-life environment. Knowledge is permanently modifiable by experience and learning: for example, it is possible to know where an object is, with minimal visual cues, due to habits (long term memory) or previous actions (short term memory). Memory generates predictions which fill in the "blanks" of the information given by the light on the retina. For example in the dark, expectations and imagination can easily give meaning to insufficient visual information. Artificial neural networks have a built-in property of learning which could provide a way of integrating individual experience into visual aids.

HOW DOES THE BRAIN RELATE IMAGES AND LANGUAGE ?

The process of scene description in the brain is the result of a global architecture relating image processing, goals, exploration, symbolic association and language production. Knowledge about this global architecture and about the functioning of its subcomponents is increasing rapidly thanks to the association of the complementary scientific fields of cognitive science:

• psychology and developmental psychology allow the decomposition of step of processing and learning; a great deal of effort is now made to interpret these steps in quantitative terms and models, with the increasing use of neural nets (Watt, 1988; Rumelhart, 1986);

• neuropsychology and brain imaging techniques allow these steps to be related to specific brain regions and groups of neurons; two new imaging techniques (Magnetic Resonance Imaging and Positon Emission Tomography) provide new insights into the comprehension of the brain subregions involved in language and image recognition (Corbetta, 1990);

• neuroscience can analyse each process in terms of circuitry and local neuronal activations. Very recent findings in the exploration of the visual areas of the cerebral cortex in primates provide a new picture of the transformation of the image (*pixels* on the retina) towards prototypes which are, in humans, the basis of a symbolic description (I see a *woman*) (Iwai, 1990).

The three main complementary processes of scene description (image processing, goals and communication) correspond to three main subregions of the cerebral cortex as seen in Fig. 1:

(1) *Visual processing* is performed by a set of cortical areas making up the visual system: each area of this system has a functional specialization: for example extraction of movements, colours and orientation of surfaces, eye movements., etc. All these specialised areas are connected to form two main *pathways* which are linked to the primary visual areas:
• The pathway formed by the areas in the temporal lobe answers the *What* questions: *What* object is fixated on the center of the retina?
• The pathway formed by areas in the parietal lobe answers the *Where* questions: *Where* is the object and where should it be moved to?

The WHAT visual system, which transforms the pixel content of the retina into a prototypical representation is better known at a fine grained level, thanks to rapidly growing experimental results on neuronal activity in the processing stream of the temporal lobe of primates. This pathway can be broken down into four processing steps ("temporal" cortex in Fig. 1):
• The first step (areas V1 and V2) provides a set of complementary filters which locally extract specific features in the image: oriented and contrasted lines, end of lines, oriented movements, color contrast, stereo 3D information (from binocular interaction).
• The second step (area V4) extracts the characteristics of local surfaces: circular or elongated shapes, spatial frequency of a simple repetitive pattern, orientation of the surface in 3D space, colours independent of lighting conditions (Gallant, 1993).
• The third step (posterior temporal areas) provides clusters of neurons which code all the main different aspects and views of a 3D object (in observer-centered co-ordinates): for example a cylinder may be circular or elongated, the surface can be lit from above or from below, etc...(Fujita, 1992).
• The fourth step (anterior temporal areas) can store the *prototypes* independently of size, orientation, position of their retinal image, independent of the point of view. Furthermore, all the relationships between prototypes can be stored (Miyashita, 1991): for example, to predict that one object is contained in another. This cortical region can integrate successive pieces of information and their spatial relationships acquired by successive exploratory eye movements (scanpath).

Through feedback connections, the result of processing at each of the four cortical steps can guide the exploration of the scene, by moving the center of gaze (the analysis of the image is much more precise in the center of the retina):
• If nothing is known, the first step can guide the center of gaze to the regions of the image with high information content (high density of contours). It is worthwhile to note that eyes, faces, hands, silhouettes, are very rich in such low level information.
• Further steps guide the successive fixation points from the partial information they have already extracted and the resulting predictions (they have learned), until recognition is complete.

(2) *Goals* correspond to the sensorimotor and cognitive programs organised in the frontal lobe of the cortex. This region answers the question: *When* to execute a specific program? Visual areas send information to the frontal cortex through feedforward connections, and the frontal cortex can reciprocally control visual processing through feedback connections. Through feedforward connections, the frontal cortex can memorise, in working memory, the different pieces of information needed to execution of the program. Through feedback connections, it can control the exploration of a scene from the question which is asked: for example, it can organise a systematic exploration to count a number of objects.

Feedback connections can select "important" and "useful" features in the scene through attentional processes depending on each goal. Parts of the brain where information is expected are far more active, as demonstrated for example in the human by brain imaging during tasks with selective attentional processes (Corbetta, 1990).

(3) *Communication* can be carried out through any couple of sensory and motor channels: visual, auditory or tactile channels to receive signals, any motor output to send a signal. A main characteristic of each channel is its capacity to transmit selective information and the speed of the communication process. Every channel can transmit either analogic signals where the spatio-temporal pattern of the signal gives direct information (for example tactile information about an object), or symbolic signals which corresponds to any set of information through a learned code (Human language with words and sentences). Brain regions which recognise and produce language are in direct interaction with areas performing visual processing and areas representing goals and sensorimotor programs (see Fig.1).

The functional specialization of cortical areas, for example the processing of images or language, is mainly due to their external connectivity (inputs and outputs) and not to their intrinsic neuronal circuits. All these areas have similar neuronal architectures, they use similar neuronal codes, they carry out the same types of neuronal operations and learning processes. In this way *images and language are represented by the same neural code in the brain.*

This simple model of cortical architecture relating image processing, goals and communication by language is shown in Fig. 1 (from Burnod, 1988): all areas have the same network of communication with other cortical areas. For the external connections, some areas form specific poles which can communicate with a specific sensory modality (visual, auditory, tactile, proprioceptive), motor system (eye, hand, leg movements), or internal drive (specific needs). Between these poles, associative areas form nodes which correlate the information coming from the different sensory and motor poles, and learn this correlation.

This process forms *multi-modal representations* of objects, people, places, actions, spatial, temporal and causal relationships, depending on the node in the cortical network. Each representation is not only activated by sensory inputs, but also by the goals of the sensorimotor and cognitive programs.

Furthermore, these representations can actively "call" any sensory or motor pole: for example, when searching for an object, an internal representation of this object can generate *active exploration* to find the appropriate configuration of pixels on the retina signalling the presence of this object.

Furthermore, sensori-motor poles and associative nodes are replicated in the two cerebral hemispheres. One hemisphere is more interested in exploring the outside world and in acquiring direct sensori-motor knowledge by storing representations, the other is more interested in acquiring knowledge through communication by storing symbols of these representations. Communication within and between hemispheres relates representations with words (for example naming people and objects, using verbs for motor actions). The main semantic components of a sentence (people, objects, locations, relations, actions) are in direct correspondence with the main cortical regions (temporal, parietal, motor...). Frontal areas (Broca's areas) in the left hemisphere can combine words into sentences to communicate all types of relations detected in a scene: for example a person carrying an object or two people shaking hands... Scene description appears as the process resulting from *a dialogue between all the cortical areas in the two cerebral hemispheres directed by goals:* a goal represented in one area calls for subgoals, sensory responses or motor actions in other areas. Such intracortical dialogue is now experimentally accessible, at a coarse grain level, thanks to the new techniques of functional imaging of the human brain.

HOW CAN AN ARTIFICIAL SYSTEM BE DESIGNED WHICH TRANSFORMS IMAGES (PIXELS FROM STEREO CAMERAS) INTO WORDS, AND WHAT ARE WE ALREADY ABLE TO DO?

Techniques of extracting information from images

Several complementary techniques are now available for the design of an artificial system which can perform scene description.

First, several techniques of *signal processing* allow the extraction of specific features in the image from the pixel content (acquired by a video camera). This analysis is composed mainly of spatial or spatiotemporal filters. Some widely used filters, such as Gabor filters which associate a spatial and a frequency analysis, are very close to the properties of neurons in the primary visual cortex. In the most efficient systems, a family of filters at several scales, such as wavelets, are applied to the image: a similar multiscale analysis is provided in the brain by retinal mapping with different receptive field sizes increasing from the center to the periphery of the retina. This filtering operation results in contour extraction which allows the separation of different zones in a scene. Orientation of these zones in 3D space is obtained by comparing the contours extracted on two images obtained by two cameras.

Recognition of an object requires the knowledge of the characteristics and structures of its 2D images in different point of views. Each object can be represented by a graph of aspects and characteristics, coded by symbols.

With this knowledge, an *expert system* with general rules can search for objects present in a scene (Brooks, 1981). Reasoning allows the elaboration of an hypothesis and the triggering of specific actions or processing to verify these hypotheses. As knowledge is not all or nothing, *fuzzy logic* allows the manipulation of variables which are not fully known. Recognition is then a progressive matching process. Since this sequential process can be very long, several systems can work in parallel and exchange their results (*distributed artificial intelligence*).

It is generally very complex to directly describe the low level content of an image with symbols (what is the appropriate pre-processing?), and to describe the structure and characteristics of an object (what is the appropriate graph?). *Artificial neural networks* have been developed to solve these two problems by analogy with the solution provided by neuronal circuits in the brain: first the information is distributed on a large number of units; second, the appropriate process is learned from examples (Rumelhart, 1986; Kohonen, 1984).

Units are connected between them to form a network such as a perceptron. The ability of such a network to process information and to recognise is given by a set of modifiable connection weights between units which shape unit activation. Several learning rules have been designed, such as local correlations between inputs and outputs (Hebb rule), a reinforcement rule and an error correcting rule (delta rule). During training sessions, examples are presented as inputs together with a desired output, given by a teacher. This output can be a symbol (represented by a position code with an all or nothing value): in this case, after learning, the network can relate each input configuration to one symbol and thus "recognise" the input (Kohonen, 1984; Pao, 1989). More generally, the output can be a continuous signal which can be learned in a similar way from a set of examples: after learning, the network is able to perform an appropriate input-output transformation. Networks with several successive layers such as multi-layer perceptrons are very useful for learning non-linear transformations with back propagation learning algorithms (Rumelhart, 1986). Neural nets have also been developed in order to process time and to generate sequences: a great deal of effort is now devoted to applying these techniques to language processing.

The use of neural nets for practical applications is limited by the number of connections which grow very rapidly with the number of input units (for example the pixels in an image). The solution which is generally proposed is an association of specialised neural nets which cooperate in order to extract useful information from a restricted region of an image. It is very interesting to note that efficient multi-network architectures are often close to the architecture of the visual system associating complementary processes, such as scanning and focusing, separation between a What and a Where pathway, etc... (Fukushima, 1988). *Biologically inspired neural nets models* provide very general solutions to relate subsymbolic and symbolic processing and to organise by learning an appropriate combination of cooperating algorithms (Marchal, 1992).

Thanks to the learning capacities of neural networks, a system continually used by the same person could memorise their personal experiences of familiar surrounding environments.

It could then automatically adapt visual processing in order to increase its efficiency, and descriptive processing in order to focus on the information which is really useful for the person. Learning capacities of neural networks could automatically adapt a general processing system to the individual habits and demands of each person.

Scene description systems for visually impaired people: processing components and feasibility

By associating these different image-processing techniques, researchers have proposed artificial systems for scene description, that is to relate the images of the environment to a symbolic description. Such systems can be operational either in limited environments or for precise goals and questions in natural environments. Thanks to the considerable progress made in computer vision, together with improvements in computer size and speed, it is possible to develop man-machine visual interfaces such as environment-sensing devices with the intent to help people with a visual impairment (Blash, 1989; Adajoui, 1992).

Most possible applications for visually impaired people can be viewed as a part of a general scheme of scene description (as shown in Fig. 2), using the same components as the brain processes (as shown in Fig. 1). A specific application is possible when all the component modules can process information in real-time.

- Goals: the main goals correspond to the basic sensorimotor and cognitive programs applied in specific environments:

- Walk: an important application for visually impaired people is to help the planning of a safe path (M. Adjouadi, 1992). The specific environment can be a street. The main subgoal is then to detect obstacles and moving object which cross the planned path.

- Explore: another application is active scanning of the environment in order to detect its main components which depend on each specific environment: a) the environment is a room, and the system gives information about the position of the larger scale 3D objects (table, door etc..); b) the environment is a computer screen or a book, and the system gives information about the content: description of the positions of texts (easy), reading of the content (much more difficult, since it has to recognise the letters).

- Search: the scanning process can be oriented to search for a class of objects in a scene. In this case, the system has to recognise the characteristics of this class of objects. Neural nets have the capacity to learn these characteristics without an a priori symbolic description. However, recognition independent of the point of view (distance, orientation, etc) is much harder.

Communication

The system has several ways of communicating with the user, as shown in Fig. 2. For example, if the goal is to walk safely, the system can provide information about an obstacle, either by emitting a warning signal if there is an obstacle just ahead, or by providing symbolic information: safe step, obstacle ahead, turn left/right.

- Fast communication, such as warning signals, is important when the system is able to detect events which can occur at any time: for example detection of relative movement towards the visual sensor. Such low-level detectors which have fast access to motor systems are common to many animal species.

- Analogic communication: vision is firstly analogic information, and some aspects can be communicated either through the tactile or the auditory channel: for example the position of a moving object and its trajectory can be translated in a binaural signal which gives a sound to the moving object. 2D information can be mapped on an array of vibro-tactile stimulators (Collins, 1976).

- Symbolic communication with words has the advantage of providing information with any level of complexity: speech synthesis systems are now currently available. Speech recognition is possible for a set of isolated words, and improves with learning from a given locutor. However, recognition of continuous speech is still very difficult and a matter of intense research.

Image processing

Real time image processing is the bottleneck for all applications, including recognition. However, applications based on low-level processing such as movement detection are now possible.

Real time low-level information processing has improved with the development of an artificial retina, which are VLSI processing in parallel the different parts of the image. Space-variant visual sensors characterised in the human retina by a resolution decreasing from the center towards the periphery are also available (Sandini, 1990). Prototypes of Specific VLSI chips detecting moving parts on a video camera and extracting the motion of objects independently of the motion of the camera have been tested and will appear in the very near future.

Systems providing 3D information about surfaces are in general composed of two cameras for stereo vision with active exploration and focusing capacities. A set of vision algorithms have been developed and successfully tested to *recover* depth perception from the disparity between the pair of stereo images provided by the two cameras (Marr, 1979). For this, images are filtered by a multi-scale analysis and a segmentation process is applied. Then, pairs of stereo images are compared with a progressive matching process which proceeds from a coarse image scale to a fine image scale, and the relative depth of the contours can be determined.

An important process for walking, safe path planning and exploring an environment is the *analysis of upright versus flat objects:* upright objects may first be obstacles to be avoided; they may also be landmarks which may help the guidance process. The processing module which signals the position and extent of upright objects exploits all the properties of vertical orientation: for example, upright objects, unlike flat objects, are not affected by the perspective effect since straight vertical edges project like on a camera. Important cues are also provided when the camera moves: changes in the image are quite different for an upright and a flat object (Adjaoui, 1992).

Recognition of objects is the most difficult problem. However, several successful algorithms have been develop to recognise specific objects linked with a sensorimotor program (Marr, 1979; Horn, 1989). For example, it is possible to recognise stereotyped 2D shapes such as letters (but not hand-written letters). It is also possible to recognise the presence of some 3D objects, such as staircases, which are critical to modify the walking program (Sakamoto, 1988): the recognition modules focus on specific charcteristics of staircase, such as a regular alternation of vertical and horizontal planes. It is also possible to eliminate irrelevant aspects of the image such as shadows: in a 2D image a shadow is easily confused with objects by segmentation processes; a module which removes shadows can use both low level information (for example, the form of histograms of grey levels), but also higher level information provided by knowledge about the orientation of the surfaces.

More general algorithms for recognition, based on learning and cooperation between algorithms, have been proposed (for example ICARE) (Marchal, 1992) and create the possibility of new developments.

REFERENCES

Adjaoui M. (1992), A man-machine vision interface for sensing the environment, *J. rehabilitation Research and Development, Vol 29 (2)*, p.h57-76.

Blash B.B., Long R.G. & Griffin-Shirley N. (1989), Results of a national survey of electronic travel aid use, *J. Vis Impairm Blindn , 83(9)*, p.449-53.

Brooks R.A. (1981), Symbolic reasoning among 3D models and 2D images, *Journal of artificial intelligence, 17*, p.235-348.

Burnod Y. (1988), *An adaptive neural network: the cerebral cortex*, Book: Masson, Prentice Hall, 400p.

Collins C.C. & Saunders F.A. (1976), Pictorial display by direct electrical stimulation of the skin, *J. Biomed Syst ,1(2)*, p.3-16.

Corbetta M., Miezin F.M., Dobmeyer S., Schulman G.L. & Petersen S.E. (1990), Attentional modulation of neural processing of shape, color and velocity in humans, *Science, 248*, p.1556-1559.

Gallant J., Braun J. & Van Essen D.C. (1993), Selectivity for polar, Hyperbolic and cartesian gratings in macaque visual cortex, *Science, 259*, p.100-103.

Fujita I., Tanaka K., Ito M. & Cheng K. (1992), Columns for visual features of objects in monkey infero-temporal cortex, *Nature, 360*, p.343 -346.

Fukushima K. (1988), Neocognitron: a hierarchical network capable of visual pattern recognition, *Neural networks, 1*, p.119-130.

Horn B.K.P. & Weldon E.J. (1988), Robust direct method for recovering motion, *Int J Comp Vision, 2*, p.51-76.

Horn B.K.P. (1989), *Shape from shading*, cambridge MIT Press.

Iwai Mishkin M. (1990), *Vision, Memory and the Temporal Lobe*, Elsevier Science Publishing Co, New York.

Kohonen (1984), Self-Organization and associative memory, Springer-Verlag.

Marchal P. & Guyot F. (1992), *MASAI: A high order connectionnist system for 3D complex image scanning*, IEEE-EMBS, Paris.

Marr D. (1979), *Vision*, Cambridge, MA:MIT Press.

Miyashita Y. & Sakai K. (1991), Neural organization for the long term memory of paired correlates, *Nature 354*, p.152-155.

Otto I., Guigon E., Grandguillaume P., Boutkhil L. & Burnod Y. (1992), Direct and Indirect Cooperation between Temporal and Parietal Networks for Invariant Visual Recognition, *Journal of Cognitive Neuroscience, 4 (1)*, p.35-57.

Pao Y.H. (1989), *Adaptive pattern recognition and neural networks*, reading MA Addison Westley.

Rumelhart D.E., Hinton G.E. & Williams R.J. (1986), Learning representations by back-propagating errors, *Nature, 323*, p.533-536.

Rumelhart D.E. & McClelland J.L. (1986), PDP models and general issues in cognitive science, In *Parallel Distributed Processing, Explorations in the microstructure of cognition*, Vol. 1: Foundations (Feldman JA, Hayes PJ, Rumelhart DE, eds), Cambridge: MIT Press, p.110-146.

Sandini G. & Tistarelli M. (1990), Vision and space-variant sensing, In *Neural networks for human and machine perception*, H. Weschler ed, Academic Press.

Sakamoto L.& Mehr E.B. (1988), A new method of stair markings for visually impaired people, *J Vis Impairm Blindn 82(1)*, p..24-7.

Watt R. (1988), *Visual processing: computational, psychophysical and cognitive research*, Hove UK: Erlbaum.

Résumé

Le langage permet de communiquer les informations sur le monde environnant obtenues par la vision. Des résultats neurobiologiques récents permettent de mieux comprendre comment le cerveau relie les images aux mots. Des efforts de recherche importants, associant traitement du signal, intelligence artificielle et réseaux de neurones formels, sont consacrés à développer des systèmes électroniques et informatiques pouvant transformer les images (les pixels de stéréo caméras) en séquences de mots fournissant des informations utiles sur l'environnement. Avec les progrès de la miniaturisation, cette recherche peut déboucher sur des interfaces donnant en temps réel des informations sur l'environnement à des personnes handicapées de la vue: par exemple, pour explorer un nouvel environnement, déterminer le chemin le plus sûr et se déplacer en évitant les dangers et les obstacles.

The Illusion of Manipulable Objects

"That you won't!" thought Alice, and, after waiting till she fancied she heard the Rabbit just under the window, she suddenly spread out her hand, and made a snatch in the air. She not get hold of anything, but she heard a little shriek and a fall, and a crash of broken glass, from whish she concluded that it was just possible it had fallen into a cucumber-fram, or something of the sort."

Lewis Carroll

Pictorial communication

Philip G. Barker

Interactive Systems Research Group, School of Computing and Mathematics, University of Teesside, Middlesbrough, Cleveland, TS1 3BA, United Kingdom

ABSTRACT

Human communication depends upon a wide range of technologies and techniques. The purpose of communication is to support the various activities in which human beings participate. People communicate with each other, and with machines, using three basic modalities: visual, tactile and sonic. Each modality can be used either individually or in combination with others in order to produce many complex methods of dialogue that often involve the multimodal exchange of information. Pictorial dialogue depends primarily upon the visual mode of communication - but not exclusively so. Because of its importance in the context of graphical user interfaces, this paper discusses the basic nature of pictorial communication and its role in the fabrication of dialogue methods for use with computer systems and various consumer products that embed some form of computer-based interactive control facility.

INTRODUCTION

The world in which we exist consists of a complex assembly of interacting systems. Each of these may have a large number of possible goal states and/or objectives that may either support or conflict with each other. In his systems map of the universe, Checkland (1972) identifies five basic types of system. These are: natural systems; transcendental systems; designed abstract systems; designed physical systems; and systems that involve human activity.

Human activity systems are important because they involve individuals (or groups of people) 'doing things' either alone, or in conjunction with each other. The activities in which people participate may involve other animate objects (such as machines and computers) in order to achieve some particular goal state.

Obviously, human activity is quite diverse - ranging, for example, from leisure to various types of academic practice and industrial/commercial endeavour. No matter what type of activity is involved, some form of communication is necessary.

Communication involves the exchange of information by meanof dialogue. As can be seen from Figure 1, people are able to communicate with each other (and with machines) using three basic 'modes' or channels of communication: visual, tactile and sonic. These channels may be used for both the transmission and receipt of information; they can also be used independently or cooperatively in order to achieve a particular communicative effect.

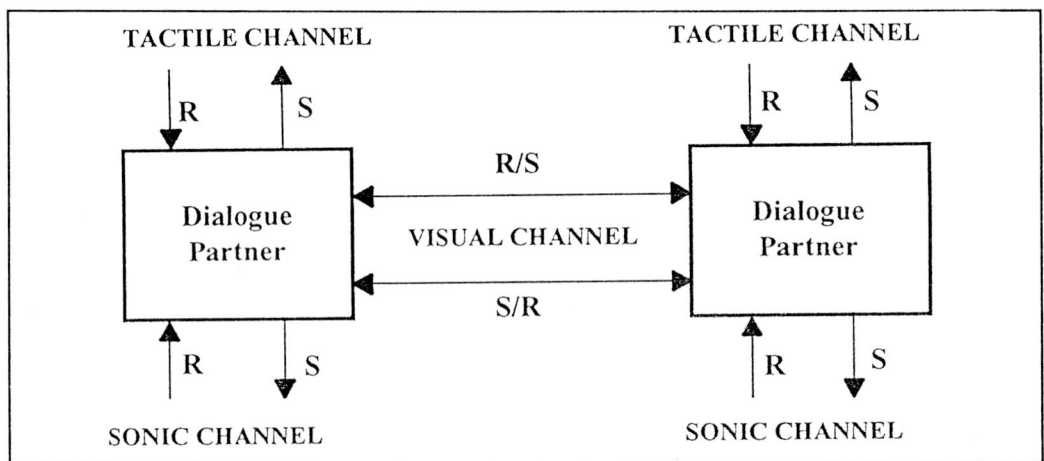

Fig. 1. Basic components of a multimodal dialogue.

Obviously, within any given situation the three modalities mentioned above can be combined in a variety of different ways in order to produce a wide range of multimodal dialogue methods. Naturally, in the case of visually impaired people the visual channel will not be available and so audio-tactile methods of communication must be used. Similarly, in the case of people who are deaf the primary mode of communication will be visio-tactile. Therefore, when one or more communication channels are not available for use (for whatever reason) the information that would normally be carried on those channels must be 'recoded' and transmitted using the other available channels. Obviously, this requirement has important implications for designers of human-computer interfaces for use by disabled people.

There are a number of approaches to designing interfaces to computer-based technology (Barker, 1989a). One approach is through the use of serial communication channels such as text and speech. An alternative method is via the use of highly parallel communication channels such as those involved in pictorial communication (Kindborg and Kollerbaur, 1987) or multimedia techniques that combine a number of channels simultaneously (Naffah and Karmouch, 1986).

We have argued elsewhere about the limitations of conventional text as a communication medium (Barker, Najah and Manji, 1987) for use in time critical applications. Our major criticism of it was its relatively slow rate of assimilation due to its inherently serial nature. Another important limitation is its lack of expressive capability For example, the printed form is unable to communicate (in an effective way) many scientific and engineering phenomena such as: flight; flow and fluid dynamics; molecular structure; weather conditions; surface and deep-lying stress patterns in objects; seismic data; radar signals; or the thermal distributions that might exist within a heat exchanger or a nuclear reactor.

The limitations of conventional text have also been discussed and debated by Waern and Rollenhagen (1983). They have made extensive studies of text readability and the potential benefits of CRT-based text compared with its paper-based equivalent. Within an interactive environment a number of methods and techniques (such as hypertext) can be employed to improve the utility of text as a communication vehicle. Unfortunately, no matter how text is improved, human-computer interface designers will always be subject to its serial nature. Consequently, for many applications its use is much less acceptable than many other forms of human-computer communication. This is particularly true in environments involving, for example, various types of visual design activity, computer-based training, medical diagnoses, image processing and manipulation and the control of complex manufacturing and production processes. In many of these situations there is a great need for more technical and cognitive bandwidth. For this reason current methods of human-computer interaction make extensive use of pictorial communication and pictorial dialogue methods.

Because of its importance with respect to the design of human-computer interfaces for future computer systems (and computer-based products) the remainder of this paper discusses the basic nature of pictorial communication and how various types of pictorial form can be used to fabricate effective and efficient human-compute interaction. The following section therefore discusses the nature of pictorial dialogue. This is followed by a section which outlines the use of graphical user interfaces within computer systems and consumer products. The final section of the paper then discusses the use of metaphors within pictorial interfaces and the growing use of virtual reality environments.

PICTORIAL DIALOGUE

In terms of human-computer interaction an interface may be regarded as a notional boundary or surface that joins together a computer and its user population. The purpose of the interface is to support the smooth flow of information that is involved in human-computer dialogue. Interfaces are usually multi-layered, often highly hybridised, sometimes intelligent, and hopefully, ergonomically sound (Barker, Najah and Manji, 1987).

Over the years human-computer interfaces have developed quite substantially in their capability. They have progressed from switches and lamps, through punched cards and paper tape to keyboards, mouse-like devices, speech-based facilities and sophisticated image analysis and production equipment. Indeed, at present, there is considerable interest in the use of pictures as a communication medium - both for the output of information to users (via computer graphics) and for its input from them (using image and picture analysis techniques). One appealing aspect of the use of pictures as a communication medium is that (in contrast to text) they offer a highly parallel mechanism for information transfer. For this reason, they provide a relatively high bandwidth communication facility. Furthermore, there is a growing volume of evidence (Barker and Skipper, 1986) to suggest that graphical communication methods based upon the use of such facilities as windows (Norman et al, 1986), icons (Gittins, 1986), comics (Kindborg and Kollerbaur, 1987), animation (Reimann, 1992) and video (Barker, 1989b) can provide powerful and efficient mechanism for the facilitation of human-computer interaction.

The general role of a pictorial interface is illustrated schematically in Figure 2. This diagram depicts the idea of human-computer communication taking place through the medium of either static images, reactive images or time varying dynamic (possibly highly animated) imagery. By reactive we mean that the content of the images changes as a result of human interaction with them. In Figure 2 the term 'multi-dimensional time varying ...' refers to the idea of having a system containing one or more screens each of which may be segmented in various ways. The information contained within each of the various screen segments may be static, reactive or time varying.

Descriptions of the relative merits of images as a communication mechanism have been presented by a number of researches (Kindborg and Kollerbaur, 1987; Barker, Najah and Manji, 1987; Larkin and Simon, 1987). Larkin and Simon, for example, have shown that pictures are useful in many problem solving situations. There is also some evidence to suggest that for certain types of cognitive activity (such as category matching) the time taken to understand pictures is less than the time needed to understand words (Potter and Faulconer, 1987). These findings would suggest two possibly important outcomes with respect to the utility of pictures as a communication resource. First that pictorial forms offer a high bandwidth mechanism of communication. Second, that pictures and images may be easier to assimilate than text and other forms of the printed word.

As we have discussed elsewhere (Barker and Manji, 1989), human computer dialogue is, in general, oscillatory in nature - each dialogue partner taking turns to transmit and receive information in a controlled, synchronised fashion. A typical scenario for a pictorial dialogue might therefore be as follows: (1) a user presents an image, an image sequence or an image referent to the computer; (2) this pictorially orientated input would embed the knowledge, information or data needed to sustain some ongoing application; (3) the computer extracts the relevant items from the input data and reacts accordingly; (4) where it is appropriate, the computer then synthesises or retrieves an image (or sequence of images); and (5) this image sequence is then presented to the user.

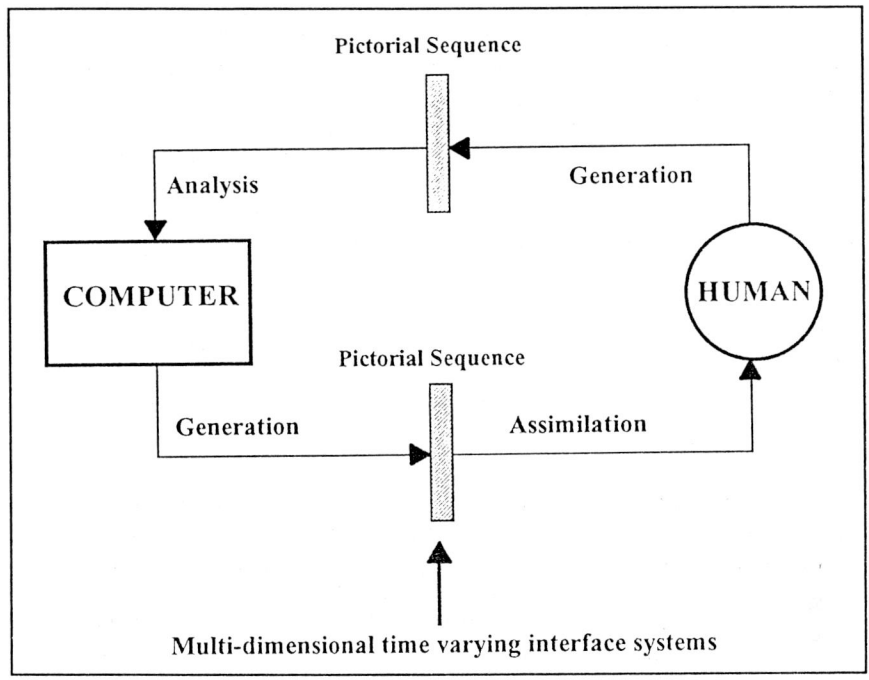

Fig. 2. The function of pictorial interfaces.

As can be seen from Figure 3 the image sequences used in a pictorial dialogue can be of three basic forms. In some situations, a single discrete time invariant image might be used. In other cases a sequence of event related pictures might be more appropriate while in other situations it might be important to use a sequence of time-related images.

Obviously, a variety of methods exist whereby a pictorial dialogue sequence could be fabricated. For example, a user might sketch (in real time) a picture on a high resolution digitiser or employ some form of sophisticated image acquisition facility (such as a colour scanner or video camera). Similarly, the computer might create an image using computational graphics or it might retrieve image segments from a video disc or CD-ROM. Through the technique of 'value added imagery' these two approaches might be combined in order to optimise the efficiency of interaction.

In the context of the output of information, the term 'visualisation' is often used to describe computational processes that analyse data and information and then present it in a pictorial format that is easily, rapidly and, hopefully, unambiguaously interpreted. For their successful realisation, visualisation processes depend critically upon the effective use of both graphics and image processing technologies.

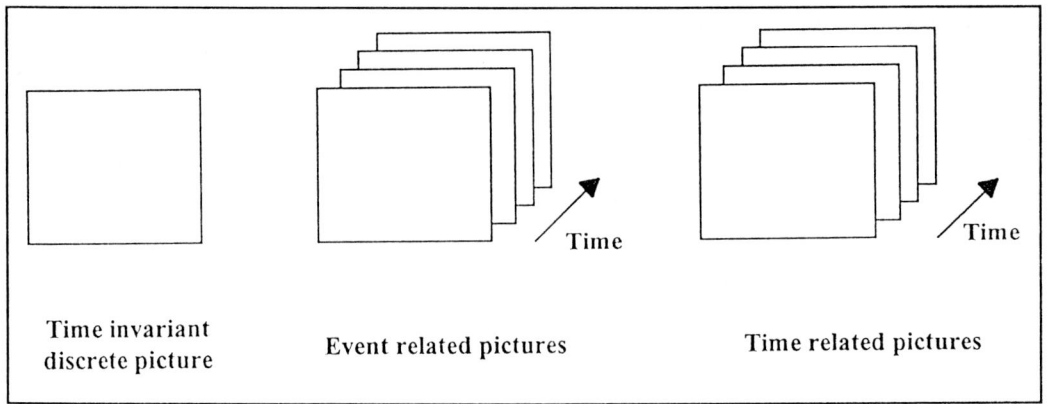

Fig. 3. Pictorial communication by means of image sequences.

Unfortunately, at present, one of the most difficult aspects of exploiting visualisation facilities is the provision of conceptual/semantic processing resources needed to (a) derive concepts from 'massed' (and possibly unstructured) data; and (b) interconvert between different representations of a concept. The mode of implementing pictorial dialogue depends critically upon the nature of the image processing equipment that is available and the characteristics of the application involved. For example, in the context of expert systems one simple way of implementing pictorial dialogue is through the use of pointing operations using either paper-based or CRT-based images (for user input) and video disc images (or images from CD-ROM) as the source of the advice that is offered during the course of the consultation (Barker, 1992).

Pictures, image segments and iconic forms can be used in a dialogue in a variety of different ways. As has been suggested above, they can constitute the only channel of communication between the computer and its user or they can form part of a multimodal message that also includes sound and text. Notice that because the sonic part of a message cannot be seen its presence is often represented through the use of a graphic icon. For example, in a multi-lingual computer-assisted learning package the user might select an appropriate accompanying audio narrative by touching an icon (such as a flag or some other national emblem) that represents the language to be used.

From what has been said above it is easy to see that within a pictorial dialogue (as in any other type of dialogue) the syntactic and semantic elements embedded within the pictorial forms that are used can be employed in order to perform a number of important functions simultaneously. In other words, the different elements contained within an image will each perform a slightly different function. Of course, this is one of the reasons why there are so many psycho-motor and cognitive benefits associated with the use of pictures.

Some of the functions that the components of a pictorial message have to perform are depicted schematically in Figure 4. The first function, and perhaps the most important, is the transmission of the message itself.

The second function is the setting of any context(s) that may need to be traken into account when the message is interpreted. Of course, the image itself is also likely to embed the rules that are to be used in its interpretation; this is the third function of the picture components. If the image is reactive then it must also contain mechanisms for controlling its own presentation and delivery. Finally, certain parts of the image might be used to communicate aesthetic and mythical values.

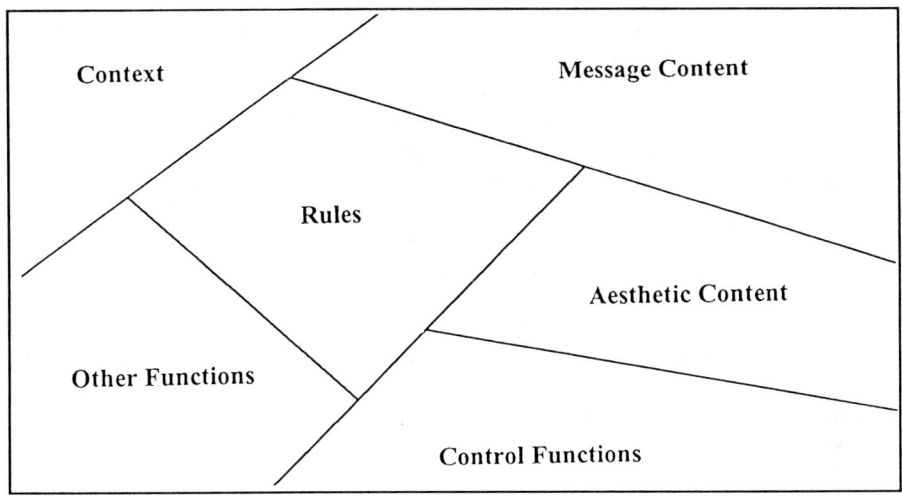

Fig. 4. *Basic functions of a reactive pictorial form.*

An example of the many functions that a pictorial multimedia interface might perform has been given by Barker and Manji (1989). The example they describe involves a paper-based graphic overlay for a concept keyboard. The paper-based concept keyboard overlay supports low resolution pointing (tactile) activity. This activity is achieved by means of finger touch operations on the surface of the overlay - which, in turn, is mounted in a suitable position on the top of a concept keyboard. Essentially, the overlay makes available pictorial/iconic menus. Depending upon where the pointing operations are made, a different context needs to be applied to their interpretation.

Thus, in the example they give, pointing operations made on the upper part of the overlay are used for the specification and selection of information. However, pointing operations made on the bottom part are used to control the presentation of the information on a CRT. The rules governing the way in which control operations can be used are contained on the pictorial syntax diagram that is embedded in the control areas of the interface.

As another example of the multiplicity of function that can be embedded within a multimodal interface, consider the use of a 'bit-mapped' screen facility. Imagine that such a high-resolution display device is fitted with a touch sensitive overlay device that is capable of responding to certain types of touch operation made upon its surface by a user.

From the interface designer's point of view a facility of this type offers a very attractive communication medium. Figure 5 depicts a typical spatial arrangement of display items within such a communication facility. In keeping with Figure 4, this diagram again brings out the idea of parallelism within an image-based multimodal message system. However, unlike the example described above, this interface, of course, is CRT-based and so can be made reactive; that is, it can be made to respond in a dynamic way to touch operations made on its surface. By 'dynamic response' we mean the ability of the interface to change its own form and appearance. Within Figure 5 the arrows that are shown denote locations within the text and/or image segments at which hypertext (or hyperimage) branches may be taken (Conklin, 1987). It is important to emphasise that the picture segment illustrated in Figure 5 could contain static, animated or video images. For example, at some particular instant in time the picture segment might contain a photo of an automobile engine. Touching a certain part of the engine might then cause a close-up view of a particular component to appear. Touching another option might cause the operation of that component (such as a fan, a pump or a motor) to be displayed - possibly accompanied by appropriate sound effects.

Most of the discussion in this section has concentrated on the use of images and pictorial forms for display purposes in order to control resources via direct manipulation. Obviously, a truly pictorial dialogue is likely to involve substantial image analysis. There are numerous reasons why images need to be analysed by automatic means. Many of these are concerned with security and surveillence, robot vision, and studies in automation.

From the point of view of pictorial dialogue one of the major objectives of image analysis is to locate and identify its syntactic and semantic elements and the relationships between them (if any exist) so that meaning can be extracted from the image. A number of ways might be used to implement the analysis depending upon the source of the image, its quality, where it is resident and whether or not the analysis is to take place in real time - that is, as it is being generated or as it is acquired. In order to illustrate the wide variety of possibilities that exist some examples will be cited. We have already mentioned the possibility of analysing sketches and the interpretation of line drawings. Another approach, (involving high degrees of parallelism) is the analysis of images that are being created in real-time from a number of different sources simultaneously. Partial image analysis can also be conducted; an example of this approach is the use of an image scanner to extract particular image segments from a paper-based image. Very often in order to extract the items of interest it is necessary to embed 'hooks' (or markers) in the picture so that the software can 'pick up' the items that it is looking for. We use this approach to study the 'meaning' in pictures that are composed from various types of icons that bear different kinds of spatial relationship with each other (Barker and Manji, 1987).

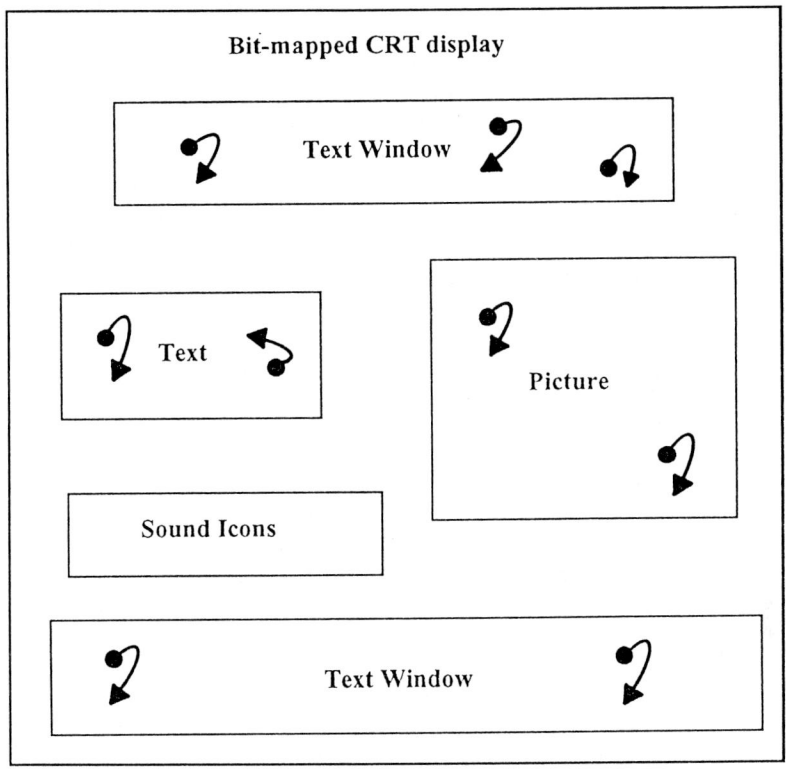

Fig. 5. Parallelism within a CRT-based image.

Obviously, a variety of different ways of generating pictorial dialogue currently exist. The approach used in any given situation is strongly influenced by the nature of the images involved, by the amount of effort needed to generate/analyse the pictorial forms that are employed and, of course, by any financial restraints that might influence the type of equipment that is used. Increasingly, there is a need to utilise low-cost equipment that is reliable, resilient and easy to use - especially where it is to be employed within consumer products. In this context, and for the reasons outlined earlier in this section, graphical user interfaces based upon simple pointing devices and high-resolution screens are becoming an extremely popular way of implementing pictorial communication. This approach to interaction is discussed in more detail in the following section.

GRAPHICAL USER INTERFACES

This section of the paper addresses three fundamental issues: the basic nature of graphical user interfaces; GUIs for use in computer systems; and the growing use of GUIs within consumer products. Some brief comments are also made about the problems GUIs present for non-sighted users.

What is a GUI?

A graphical user interface is essentially a sequence of one or more CRT-based 'scenes' that embed various types of reactive graphical object with which a user can interact either directly (by means of touch operations) or indirectly by means of a screen-based pointer (cursor). When a cursor is involved its screen position is usually controlled by an appropriate direct manipulation device such as a mouse, a roller-controller, a thumbstick controller or a joystick (Barker, 1989a). In normal use, such devices obviously depend upon the availability of a visual channel of communication from the computer to the user and a sonic or tactile channel from the user to the computer (see Fig. 1). A sighted person can thus interact with a screen-based object by pointing at it (by moving the cursor onto the object of interest) and then activating it by pressing an 'action button' on the pointing device. Subsequent interaction may then involve further selection, the movement of an object around the screen or the entry of textual or graphical information.

The types of object that can appear within a CRT-based scene can include: windows, menu bars, dialogue boxes, icons, control bars, control buttons and various sorts of 'decorative' material. Three of the most interesting and important types of screen-based object within a GUI are icons, menus and windows.

Icons are 'stamp sized' pictorial representations of objects, system resources and/or system states; they can be either reactive or unreactive. Due to the technological improvements that have taken place in computer hardware and software over the last few years (particularly with respect to graphics handling) the use of icons within graphical user interfaces has become extremely popular. The 'hour glass' and 'trash can', for instance, are now familiar examples to most Windows and Macintosh users. Indeed, as a result of this popularity a number of different types of icon have now been developed. Currently, some of the most popular of the new developments are 'picons', 'micons' and 'earcons'. Picons are essentially icons that embed a picture (as opposed to a symbol). Similarly, micons are composed of moving pictures or video clips. Earcons, or auditory icons, are based upon the use of sounds and are usually embedded in sonic sequences (Gaver, 1989).

Menus are reactive objects that provide a user with a list of graphically or textually labelled control options to facilitate use of an application system. In some situations (especially where blind users are involved) menus may take the form of an audio narration that can be 'interrupted' at an appropriate point by the user. Obviously, menus can take a variety of different forms and may possess a range of characteristics.

For example, they can be located at various places on the screen and can assume a variety of different shapes and spatial orientations. Menus can be of a static or dynamic nature (such as: pull-down, pop-up, pop-out, and so on) and may remain invisible until they are needed. In some situations menus can be structurally complex if they consist of a multi-level structure. Usually, for most menu options keyboard 'short-cuts' or 'accelerator' keys are also available.

Windows are more complex objects than icons and menus. They can be used for a multiplicity of different purposes - for example, the display of text, static pictures, animations and moving pictures (such as partial-screen motion video). Windows can also embed icons and, in some cases, they can be 'iconised' to form a group icon. Depending upon the size of the windows that are used in any given situation, a CRT screen can simultaneously display many windows. As can be seen from Figure 6, these can be non-overlapping discrete entities (as shown in the left-hand side of the diagram) or overlapping objects (as illustrated in the right-hand side of the figure). Obviously, the complexity of the window arrangement within any given graphical scene will significantly influence the ease with which it can be analysed, interpreted and employed - this is particularly so in the case of visually impaired users (in this situation suitable 'translation' mechanisms would be needed).

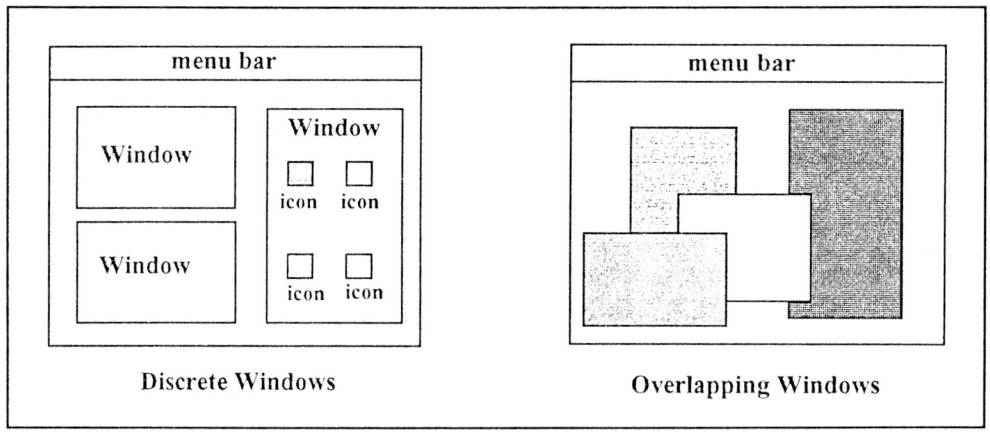

Fig. 6. Window formats and embedded icons.

GUIs for Computer Use

Unfortunately, as hinted above, the growing use of GUIs within computer systems means that non-sighted users are finding it increasingly difficult to use such interfaces and the software that they embed. In order to solve this problem some method of converting the visual information embedded in a GUI into audio-tactile form must be found. Research into methods of solving this problem is well-documented in the literature (Schwerdtfeger, 1991; Boyd et al, 1990; Frank, 1992; Petrie and Gill, 1992; Pugh et al, 1992).

Graphical user interfaces for computer use fall into two broad categories: those supplied by computer manufacturers and software supliers; and those developed by computer users using interface development kits.

Examples of fairly well-known, popular GUIs that run within personal computer (PC) environments include Microsoft's Windows products (for IBM PCs) and the desktop GUI that is used extensively in Apple Macintosh computers.

Other examples of commercially available software products that embed graphical user interfaces include PROPI (a graphical front-end to the PC/PILOT system) and Authorware Professional. Both of these are popular courseware authoring tools that are used for developing computer-based training material. Obviously, commercially available GUIs such as these do not have any inherent features that make them suitable for easy translation into a form that non-sighted users can employ.

Because of the availability of GUI toolkits, end-users of computer systems are making increasing use of graphical interface techniques within their own products. Obviously, in situations such as this, the interface designer is in a good position to influence the final shape and form of the GUI that is produced. This means that where there is a need to make the interface 'translatable' for visually impaired users, interface designers can significantly influence system design in a way that makes its subsequent translation into audio form an easier task. However, in order to make this approach effective, appropriate interface design guidelines are needed. At present, few (if any) guidelines exist to aid GUI designers to produce translatable interfaces. Considerable research is therefore needed within this area.

GUIs within Consumer Products

Increasingly, graphical user interfaces are becoming an important part of many different kinds of consumer product for use in home environments. Unfortunately, the growing use of such interfaces often reduces product accessibility for those who are visually impaired. As an illustration of the trend towards the use of a GUI within consumer products we need only consider the types of technology that is currently being used for playing digital audio (DA) from compact disc (CD).

The conventional approach to end-user control of compact disc digital audio (CD-DA) material is through the use of a CD player that embeds a simple LCD (for information read-out purposes) and an array of facia buttons (for control.purposes). In contrast, the latest 'compact disc interactive' (CD-I) equipment from Philips Electronics (which plays CD-DA as a subset of its overall functionality) uses a screen-based GUI (displayed on a TV screen) and a roller-controller (or a thumbstick device) to control the position of an on-screen cursor. Details of CD-I equipment are well-documented in the literature (Bruno, 1987; Preston, 1988; Philips IMS, 1992a; 1992b; 1992c). The basic system is illustrated schematically in Figure 7.

The configuration shown in this diagram consists of a standard CD-I player, a TV set for the display of visual material, a set of loudspeakers for playing stereo and mono sound and a roller-controller. The roller-controller is a pointing device that is used to control the position of the on-screen CD-I pointer. It has two action buttons - labelled B1 and B2 in the figure. The roller-controller plugs directly into the CD-I player.

The Philips CD-I equipment can be used to play conventional CD audio discs, CD+Graphics discs, CD-I titles and Photo CD discs. Each type of disc has its own characteristic GUI that is embedded within a proprietory user interface management system (UIMS).

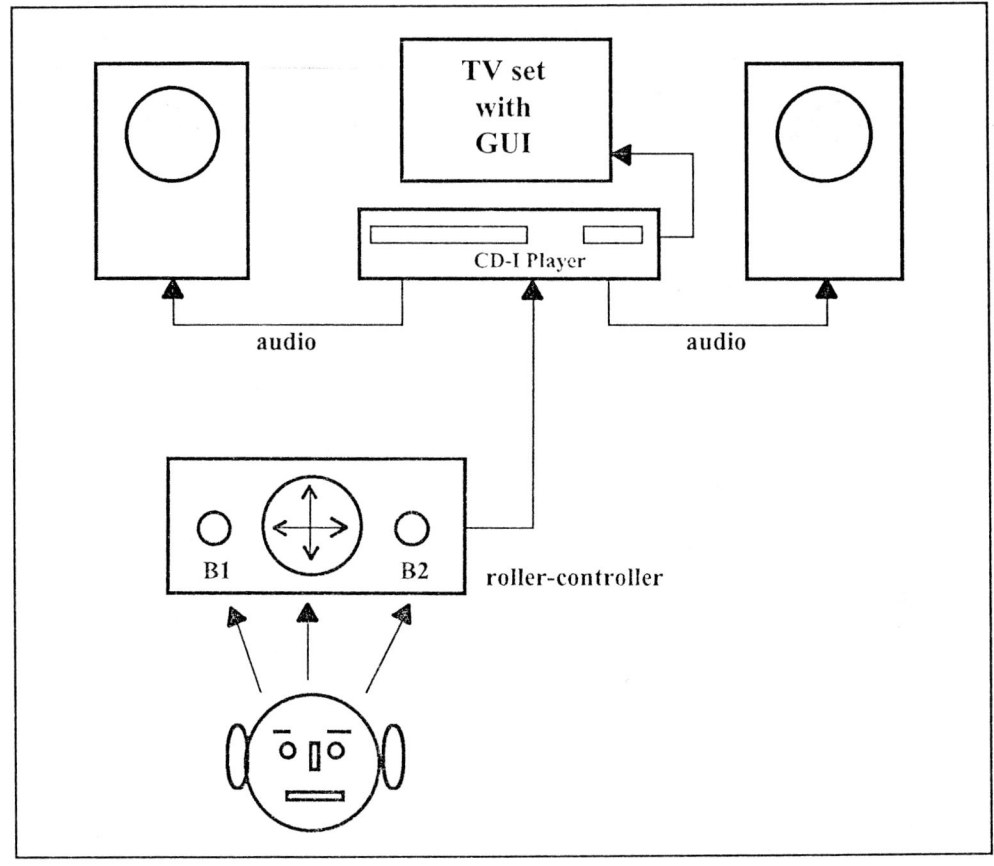

Fig. 7. The compact disc - interactive (CD-1) environment.

As an example of a consumer orientated GUI we shall consider the particular one that is used for controlling CD-DA. There is no doubt that the graphical user interface for controlling the presentation of CD-DA discs through the CD-I equipment undoubtedly improves the quality of the end-user interface (for sighted users).

It does this by: (a) making the system easier to use; and (b) improving the overall functionality that is available to the user. The functionality that is embedded within the CD-DA GUI contains four basic scenes which we refer to as: top-level control; 'FTS' programming; simulated keyboard; and memory status.

The basic interface functions contained within the CD-DA GUI allow audio discs to be played, stopped and restarted (from the beginning) and paused and restarted (from the pause point). The individual tracks on the CD can be directly accessed using a dynamic visual numeric index (1, 2, 3, ...) by means of point-and-click operations.

It is also possible to program a favourite track selection (FTS) which can be named and then stored within the system's memory bank. The naming of the FTS is achieved using a simulated on-screen keyboard by means of point-and-click operations. Once a FTS has been created and stored it can be called up at any time in order to control the presentation of subsequent audio material. The FTS button also allows control to be passed back to 'full access' level - if and when this is needed. At any time after it has been stored, the FTS associated with a given CD-DA disc can be re-programmed or deleted when it is no longer needed.

From what has been said above, it is easy to see that the application of GUI techniques in consumer products can make them much easier to use - for sighted users. Unfortunately, however, their use presents many difficult problems for non-sighted users.

METAPHORS IN GRAPHICAL USER INTERFACES

Metaphors are an important aspect of human-computer interface design and use (Richards et al, 1992; Carroll, Mack and Kellogg, 1988). They are important for two basic reasons. First, they can be used to reduce the overall conceptual complexity of a computer application by likening it to something else that probably already exists within a user's cognitive framework. Second, they can act as powerful design aids during the actual construction of a computer-based application and its set of end-user interfaces.

In order to use a computer-based application in an effective way it is important that users acquire an appropriate cognitive model relating to that application. The metaphors (and 'myths') that are embedded (either explicitly or implicitly) in an end-user interface to an application are powerful tools for the development of the cognitive and conceptual models that are needed in order to use that application (Rubenstein and Hersh, 1984).

A range of different types of metaphor have been used to develop computer-based products - such as the desktop metaphor and metaphors involving the concepts of travel, books, libraries, museums, rooms, and so on. In much of our work we have found that book metaphors have been an extremely useful asset (Barker, 1991).

Because of their importance we believe that metaphors should be used from the earliest specification and design phases of an application development project. Indeed, many system development methodologies now include metaphor design in their early conceptualisation stage.

Of course, in situations where appropriate metaphors can be found and which provide precise system views, interfaces of significant effectiveness can be developed. The greater the precision of the system image produced by a metaphor - the less likely it is that ambiguous or erroneous images of the system will occur.

Obviously, metaphors chosen for use in end-user interfaces must be easy to represent. Therefore, it is important that distinctive images (which are representative of the desired functionality) can be created in a limited presentation area.

For example, the book metaphor must, through its metaphorical representation, relay to a user the image of: a book; a series of pages; a front cover; a contents list; and so on (Barker, 1991). Using this simple example it is easy to see how a metaphor can provide a framework for the design of the icons that are to be used in a given pictorial interface system.

Another important aspect of pictorial interface design is 'understandability'. Obviously, the interface set that is derived from any given metaphor must be a suitable one for the target end-user population that is to use it. If users fail to understand the implications of the metaphor (either consciously or unconsciously) then it will be of little value. This consideration becomes particularly critical in pictorial interfaces that are intended for international use -where it is even more difficult to identify a useful metaphor.

Extensibility is another aspect of the use of powerful metaphors in pictorial interface design. Indeed, the use of a good metaphor can often provide many useful ideas for improving an existing design. Extensions to an existing system may be suggested by properties of the metaphor which are appropriate to the system being designed. In addition, the parts of the metaphor which go beyond the current implementation can provide for additional functionality in the future.

With the complexity and high functionality which is a key aspect of many modern applications, a single metaphor may not support all the facilities which are needed. In such circumstances multiple metaphors can be used (Richards et al, 1992). One example could be a book and a travel metaphor that are embedded within an implementation of a hypermedia electronic book. This approach provides a user with several strategies for navigating through and retrieving information from a complex hypermedia knowledge corpus.

An area which can have a critical impact on the usability of future iconic interfaces is the idea of standards. Sets of recommended, tried and tested icons, based upon particularly useful, and culturally relatively common metaphors, could be produced. When such a metaphor is appropriate for a particular application, these tried and tested icons can be 'taken off the shelf' and used. In this way, similar functionality across a wide range of applications can be represented by a standard icon. Further, sets of standard icons would be used in different applications based upon the same metaphor. In this way, user experience would be highly transportable between different computer applications.

Sometimes, the meaning of icons used to support a particular metaphor can be ambiguous and difficult to decode unless considerable care is taken in designing them. Therefore, one of the principle methods used for enhancing the meaning of icons is to use multiple modality. Text is the form of augmentation that is most frequently used to support the meaning of an icon. Two basic types of textual support can be used: permanent (or static) labels; and dynamic labels. Permanent labels are usually found attached to the base of an icon - as can be seen in many of those used in both the Apple Macintosh and the Microsoft Windows desktop metaphors.

Dynamic labels are less common; in this case the textual augmentation only appears once the mouse pointer is moved over its host icon. As well as textual augmentation, audio augmentation may also take place.

Of course, serious problems can arise from the use of textual and audio augmentation - particularly, with respect to international interface designs. Obviously, if an interface is intended for international use then any textual labels which have been attached to it must be dynamically switchable between the target languages.

An Example

The use of metaphors in the design of conventional computer products is quite well-established (Carroll, Mack and Kellogg, 1988). Undoubtedly, in this context one of the most well-known metaphors is the 'desktop' metaphor that underlies many Macintosh products. The book metaphor is also quite well known as are the travel metaphors that are used for navigating through complex hypermedia knowledge corpora.

Metaphors are also starting to be used in interactive products intended for the consumer market. The way in which they are used will be illustrated by means of an example choosen from the rapidly expanding range of commercially available products designed to run on the Philips' CD-I equipment illustrated in Figure 7. The example that has been selected for discussion is 'Treasures of the Smithsonian'.

'Treasures of the Smithsonian' is a CD-I title produced by the Smithsonian Institute. The disc itself is a standard 12 cm CD-ROM disc which stores a large amount of high-quality digital audio-visual material. Through the use of a museum metaphor this CD-I title allows users to explore the highlights of the 13 museums and the National Zoo which make up this famous American institution. The end-user interface allows users to browse through multiple subject areas and museums, explore links between objects and even 'walk around' statues.

As with many modern museums, 'Treasures of the Smithsonian' provides a wide range of additional information in a variety of media forms. For instance, most museums provide a plaque containing textual information about each exhibit. In addition, some museums also provide audio facilities which allow visitors to access multi-lingual audio narrations which provide further information. In a similar fashion, 'Treasures of the Smithsonian' also provides multiple channels of audio-visual information provision.

When 'entering the Smithsonian', within the first two screens users are immediately exposed to all the icon types (although not all the icons) which are used within the application. The first type of icon to be encountered is the dynamic 'mixed form' icon. When first viewed, icons in this class appear to be of the more traditional single graphic type. However, when the cursor is moved over an icon of this type it changes its form - from graphic to textual. This transition is used to provide further information about the individual function of the icon.

The second screen, which projects the myth of being in the entrance hall of the museum, uses picture icons to provide access mechanisms to the exhibits in the museum. The picons embedded in the mythical museum entrance are not made explicitly obvious to users until the screen cursor is moved into one of their areas of definition.

That is, each picon appears to be just a part of the entrance hall until the cursor is moved within its physical boundary. When this happens the reactive area of the host picon then becomes highlighted, thus making it visible as an actual icon. Once again, textual augmentation takes place in order to provide further information about the functional nature of the picon that has been selected.

One of the advantages of picons over traditional icons is their communicative power. In situations where only very few icons are required, and their size will not interfere with the working area, picons can be used to good effect. In the entrance hall of the museum the picons themselves therefore act as a major part of the communication strategy. This means that rather than detracting from the working area, the picons form an integral component of the entrance hall myth associated with the museum metaphor.

In addition to using a museum metaphor (the primary metaphor), 'Treasures of the Smithsonian' also embeds secondary and tertiary metaphors. For example, a 'guided tour' facility is provided and details of the thirty options available are presented in the form of a simple 'catalogue' through which users can browse. Some examples of the theme options that a user may choose from include: The Age of Steam; Art about Art; Born to Rule; Dreams and Visions; Going in Circles; Making Music; Thinking Machines; and so on. A user can thus select a theme of interest and then be guided through the collection of exhibits that make up that theme.

As was suggested above, metaphors are now being used quite extensively in an ever increasing range of interactive computer-based products intended for the mass consumer market. Typical consumer products of this sort include: sophisticated games; information resources; educational material; entertainment titles; leisure items; and so on. The metaphors that are used within these products depend very much for their implementation upon pictorial communication methods that embed sophisticated graphical user interfaces for navigation and control purposes.

FUTURE POSSIBILITIES - REAL OR VIRTUAL?

In one form or another computer systems are playing an increasingly important part in our lives. More and more we are placed in situations where we need to communicate with a computer system or with other people by means of some form of computer facility. Because of the efficiency and effectiveness of pictorial communication methods they are now being used as a basis for human-computer dialogue in a wide variety of different contexts.

The complexity of the pictorial material that is used in human-computer dialogues varies considerably - depending upon their purpose and intent. The use of icons, pictographic languages and high quality static images is now well-established.

Animation techniques, 3-D computer graphics and digital motion video are also becoming very popular. Indeed, the use of motion video (either full-screen or partial-screen) is now an important resource in many kinds of computer application - such as computer-based training, simulations, security and surveillance, telepresence, and so on.

Obviously, the use of TV quality motion video pictures within a human-computer interface enables very high levels of 'photo-realism' to be attained. Of course, photo-realism within an interface can also be achieved by means of a conventional 35 mm camera. Kodak's Photo-CD, for example, enables conventional photographs to be transferred to CD. They can then be displayed on the screen of a computer or on a TV. Obviously, the ability to manipulate photo-realistic images in this way now makes possible the creation of many new types of computer application in which pictorial interfaces play an important role - such as electronic books, interactive catalogues, training manuals with moving pictures, and so on.

One important area that is rapidly developing as a consequence of the use of animation techniques, 3-D computer graphics and high-quality digital video within the interface domain is 'virtual reality' (Barker, 1993; Helsel and Paris, 1991; Rheingold, 1991). Depending upon the way in which it is implemented, virtual reality (VR) can take a variety of different forms - for example, telepresence, graphic simulations, surrogations, shared cyberspaces, and so on. The important role that graphical techniques and pictorial communication play within a VR environment is illustrated schematically in Figure 8.

Undoubtedly, virtual reality has become an extremely important mechanism for providing highly interactive learning and training environments. Many people have described virtual reality as the 'ultimate multimedia experience'. Undoubtedly, the power of VR lies in its ability to create powerful multimedia visualisation techniques that offer a range of mechanisms by which new multi-sensory experiences can be made available through the use of pictorial, tactile and gestural communication methods.

A VR system is a sophisticated multimedia environment in which users are exposed to, and can participate in, surrogate tacto-audio-visual experiences. These experiences are created by means of a computer system to which is attached special types of peripheral device (such as a data glove, a body suit or a head-mounted display); these peripherals enable users to see and interact with the real and artificial objects that exist within a given interaction environment. The interaction environment available to the 'players' within a virtual reality is often called a 'cyberspace'. Cyberspaces may be of two basic types: local or remote. A local cyberspace exists only within the 'deck' that creates it (a deck is essentially a three-dimensional workstation). A remote cyberspace has to be accessed by means of suitable telecommunications links. Cyberspaces can be designed for use by individuals or for group use - the latter are referred to as shared cyberspaces.

VR technologies will undoubtedly have a significant impact over the next decade in terms of the potential they can bring within areas such as learning, new kinds of sensory and cognitive experience, new kinds of communication aid, training facilities and various kinds of spin-off development.

Obviously, one of the attractive features of VR as a learning and training tool is its ability to display objects and situations that are not normally visible to humans, and to enable humans to interact with them - for example, by reaching out to 'touch' the atoms of a complex molecule.

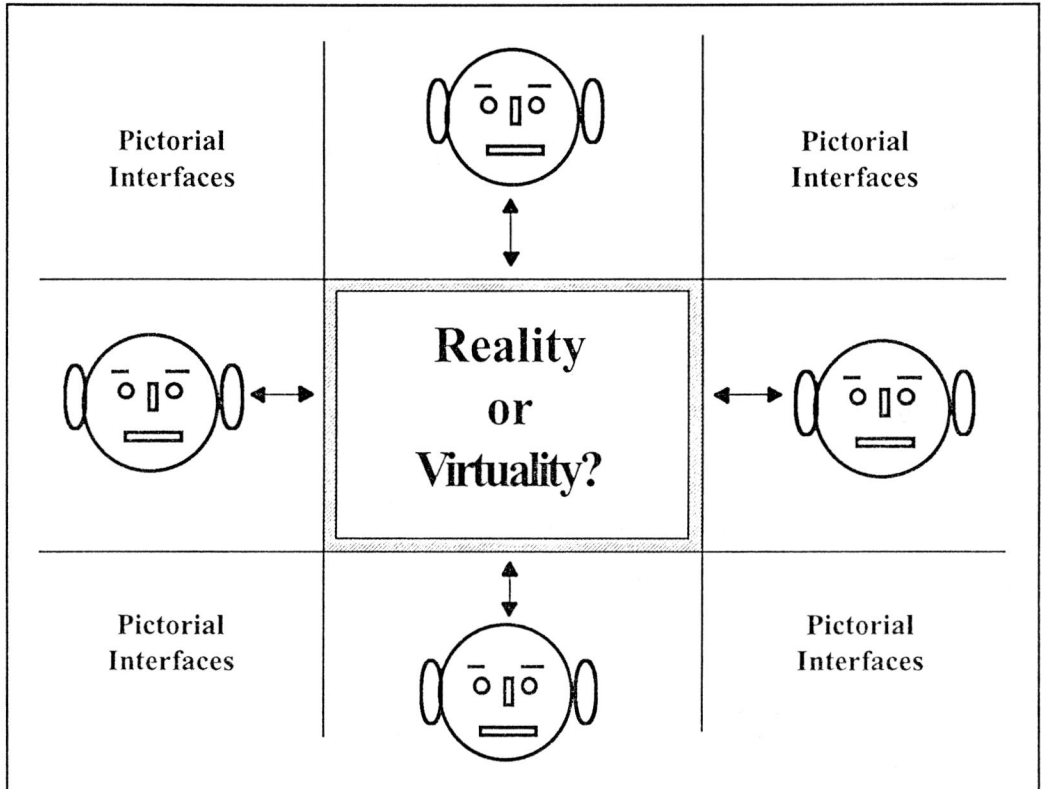

Fig. 8. The role of pictorial communication in creating virtual reality environment.

Just as easily, it could convert a wheel-chair into a vehicle capable of exploring virtual safari parks or cities anywhere in the world. Equally, because they are based on sophisticated simulations, VR systems also enable us to explore learning domains by means of 'what if' experiments - the results of which will stimulate the development of cognitive models and mental skills that could be applied in many different situations. Future VR systems will undoubtedly offer many exciting ways of learning - of course, including experiential learning.

CONCLUSION

Of the three modalities used to support human/human and human/computer interaction the visual mode is undoubtedly the most powerful. Through the mechanism of vision we are able to read, touch, watch and observe events that are taking place in both the real world and the many artificial worlds that can be created by means of computer systems. Obviously, our visual system plays an extremely important part in virtually all the normal communication processes in which we participate.

Languages that are based upon visual communication methods are therefore both varied and complex. This paper has attempted to describe the nature of pictorial communication It has also tried to illustrate some of the ways in which this method of communication is currently being used to facilitate human-computer interaction. It has also hinted at some of the ways in which pictorial communication might be used in the future in order to create sophisticated interactive three-dimensional human-computer interfaces. Within such interfaces, through the use of photo-realism and natural response times, it will be difficult for users to distinguish between reality and virtuality.

REFERENCES

Barker P.G. (1989 a), *Basic Principles of Human-Computer Interface Design*, London, Century-Hutchinson.

Barker P.G. (1989 b), *Multimedia Computer-Assisted Learning*, Kogan Page, London.

Barker P.G. (1991), Electronic Books, *Special Edition of Educational and Training Technology International*, 28(4), p.269-368.

Barker P.G. (1992), Using Pictures in Expert Systems, *Engineering Applications of Artificial Intelligence*, 5(4), p.329-344.

Barker P.G. (1993), Virtual Reality - Theoretical Basis, Practical Applications, *Journal of the Association of Learning Technology*, 1(1), in press.

Barker P.G. & Manji K.A. (1987), Pictorial Knowledge Bases, In *Proceedings of the British Computer Society HCI '87 Conference, University of Exeter*, Cambridge University Press, Cambridge, UK, 7-11 September 1987, p.161-173.

Barker P.G. & Manji K.A. (1989), Pictorial Dialogue Methods, *International Journal of Man-Machine Studies*, 31, p.323-347.

Barker P.G., Najah M. & Manji K.A. (1987), Pictorial communication with Computers, *International Journal of Man-Machine Studies*, 27, p.315-336.

Barker P.G. & Skipper T.J. (1986), A Practical Introduction to Authoring for Computer-Assisted Instruction - Part 7: Graphic Support, *British Journal of Educational Technology*, 17(3), p.194-212.

Boyd L.H., Boyd W.L. & Vanderheiden G.C. (1990), The Graphical User Interface: Crisis, Danger and Opportunity, *Journal of Visual Impairment and Blindness, 84*, p. 496-502.

Bruno R. (1987), Making Compact Discs Interactive, *IEEE Spectrum, 24(11),,* p. 40-45.

Carroll J.M., Mack R.L. & Kellogg W.A. (1988), Interface Metaphors and User Interface Design, In *Handbook of Human-Computer Interaction*, edited by H. Helander, Elsevier Science Publishers B.V. (North Holland), Amsterdam, The Netherlands, p.67-85.

Checkand P.B. (1972), A Systems Map of the Universe, In *Systems Behaviour*, edited by J. Beishon and G, Peters, Open University Press, London, UK, p.50-55.

Conklin J. (1987), Hypertext: an Introduction and Survey, *IEEE Computer, 20(9),,* p.17-41.

Frank J. (1992), *Access to Graphic User-Interfaces for the Blind: a Progress Report on a Seemingly Paradoxical Project*, Oberhausen-Rheinhausen, Germany: Frank Audiodata.

Gaver W.W. (1989), The Sonic Finder: an Interface that uses Auditory Icons, *Human-Computer Interaction*, 4, p.67-94.

Gittins D. (1986), Icon-based Human-Computer Interaction, *International Journal of Man-Machine Studies*, 24, p.519-543.

Helsel S.K. & Paris J.P. (1991), *Virtual Reality - Theory, Practice and Promise*, Meckler, Westport, CT, USA.

Kindborg M. & Kollerbaur A. (1987), Visual Languages and Human Computer-Interaction, In *Proceedings of the British Computer Society HCI '87 Conference, University of Exeter*, Cambridge University Press, Cambridge, UK, 7-11 September 1987, p.175-187.

Larkin J.H. & Simon H.A. (1987), Why a Picture is (sometimes) Worth Ten Thousand Words, *Cognitive Science*, 11, p.65-99.

Naffah N. & Karmouch A. (1986), Agora - an Experiment in Multimedia Message Systems, *IEEE Computer, 19(5)*, p.56-66.

Norman K.L., Weldon L.J. & Shneiderman B. (1986), Cognitive Layouts of Windows and Multiple Screens for User Interfaces, *International Journal of Man-Machine Studies*, 25, p.229-248.

Petrie H. & Gill J. (1992), Current Research on Access to Graphical User Interfaces for Visually Disabled Computer Users, To appear in *'European Journal of Special Needs Education'*.

Philips IMS. (1992 a), *Introducing CD-I*, Wokingham, England, UK: Addison-Wesley Publishing Company.

Philips IMS. (1992 b), *The CD-I Design Handbook*, Wokingham, England, UK: Addison-Wesley Publishing Company.

Philips IMS. (1992 c), *The CD-I Production Handbook*, Wokingham, England, UK: Addison-Wesley Publishing Company.

Preston J.M. (1988), *Compact Disc - Interactive: a Designer's Overview*, Deventer, The Netherlands: Kluwer Technical Books.

Pugh K., Harness S., Sherkat N. & Whitrow R. (1992), Icon Recognition for Providing Access to WIMP Interfaces for the Blind and Partially Sighted, *Paper presented at the First International Conference on Iconic Communication, University of Brighton, UK*, 11-12 December 1992.

Potter M.C. & Faulconer B.A. (1975), Time to Understand Pictures and Words, *Nature, 253*, p.437-438.

Reimann G. (1992), Animation in Electronic Books, *Outline PhD Proposal, Interactive Systems Research Group, School of Computing and Mathematics, University of Teesside*, Cleveland, UK.

Rheingold H. (1991), *Virtual Reality*, Secker and Warburg, London.

Richards S., Barker P.G., Banerji A.K., Lamont C. & Manji K.A. (1992), The Use of Metaphors in Iconic Interface Design, *Paper presented at the First International Workshop on Iconic Communication, University of Brighton*, 11th-12th December 1992.

Rubenstein R. & Hersh H. (1984), *The Human Factor - Designing Computer Systems for People*, Digital Press, Burlington, MA, USA.

Schwerdtfeger R.S. (1991), Making the GUI Talk, *BYTE, 16(13)*, p.118-128.

Wearn Y. & Rollenhagen C. (1983), Reading Text from Visual Display Units (VDUs), *International Journal of Man-Machine Studies, 18*, p.441-465.

Résumé

La communication homme-homme dépend d'une grande variété de technologies et de techniques. Son but est de faciliter les activités très diverses auxquels participent les êtres humains. Que le dialogue se déroule directement avec une personne, ou par l'intermédiaire d'une machine, il peut emprunter trois modalités principales, visuelle, tactile et auditive, chacune d'elle pouvant être utilisée seule ou en combinaison avec les autres. Les échanges prennent des formes variées, complexes et le plus souvent multimodales.

La communication pictographique est fortement liée par sa nature même à la modalité visuelle, mais peut aussi faire intervenir d'autres sens. Ce type particulier de communication joue un rôle essentiel dans le contexte des interfaces en mode graphique. Cet article en rappelle les principes de base et les principales caractéristiques, ainsi que son potentiel pour la réalisation de systèmes d'interface destinés à faciliter l'utilisation de l'ordinateur aussi bien que de produits technologiques de grande diffusion.

Direct manipulation of data

Agnès Roby-Brami

INSERM, Groupe CREARE, Neurosciences et Modélisation, Institut des Neurosciences, Université Pierre-et-Marie-Curie, 9, quai Saint-Bernard, 75252 Paris Cedex 05, France

ABSTRACT

Manipulation of objects in the real world implies that people have acquired the necessary sensori-motor representations through their actions on the world. This paper reviews physiological and psycho-physiological evidence demonstrating the anticipatory control of goal-directed movements and the mechanisms of learning. These data are used to interpret sensory-motor interactions within direct manipulation interfaces. The place of gestures in man-machine interactions is reviewed for the different peripheral devices and some implications for people with sensory or motor disabilities are underlined.

INTRODUCTION

Object oriented human computer interfaces make use of metaphors of the real world in order to facilitate interactions and make them more intuitive (Ziegler and Fehnrich, 1990). Visual metaphors or icons are the most widely used, for example those used in the MacIntosh desk. They may represent data (papersheets, folders ...), tools (handles of windows, brushes in drawing programs...) or even complex commands (buttons, icons representing programs). The interface includes not only icons but also several actions, consistent with the metaphor of the interface, that may be applied to the icons. Gestures are an integral part of human computer interactions and operations on icons are often carried out with a pointing device such as a mouse or by direct designation (on a touch sensitive screen for example). The coding of an action on the application usually implies a complex sequence of gestural commands. For example "delete a file" is coded as "displace the mouse cursor until it reaches the icon corresponding to the data file, select it by pressing the mouse button, drag it up to the paperbasket icon, release the button when the paperbasket is selected". The objects of the interactive interfaces are such that all the actions which change their state are signalled to the users by sensory feedback. Visual feedback (the selection of a file induces a change of the icon color) may be associated with auditory feedback (clicks, sounds). Tactile and proprioceptive feedback are used implicitly during gestural commands (for example, users have tactile sensation of contact and proprioceptive perception of the position of their figertips when acting on a touch sensitive screen).

This type of feedback has been explicitly implemented in some recent laboratory prototypes. The role of gestural interactions within the human-computer interface will probably increase in the near future with the development of multimodal interactions and virtual reality. This trend is certainly encouraging for visually impaired users who may rely on haptic sensations related to active touching during the gestural commands in order to alleviate the need for visual communication.

The aim of this paper is to review some applications of gestural commands in human computer interactions in the light of recent experimental data in the real world. The focus will be on recent neurophysiological interpretations of sensorimotor co-ordination during manipulative actions that may shed light on mechanisms involved in the construction of representations related to motor learning.

INTERACTING WITH THE REAL WORLD

Perception and action cycles

Recent theoretical trends are now bridging the gap between ideas from cognitive and developmental psychology and neural sensori-motor mechanisms. The acquisition of perceptual representations is linked to the acquisition of motor schemas (or programs) via the action-perception cycle. Subject' exploration of the world is directed by anticipatory perceptual schemas and the information picked up during the exploration modifies the perceiver's anticipation. The construction of representations has been compared to an adaptive controller process directed by the comparison of the expected and the actual perceptual consequences of the action (Arbib, 1981).

Adaptive mechanisms may be compared with the properties of parallel distributed processing of formal neurons (Rumelhart & Mc Clelland 1986). In addition, models using biologically compatible formal neurons may lead to further advances in the comprehension of perception and action cycles (Burnod 1988).

This perspective, concerning "the continuous and spontaneous changing state of the sensori-motor system" (Newell, 1992), unifies the fields of motor control, motor skill acquisition and development.

Movement and representations

Motor control implies that subjects have acquired, through experience, both motor schemas or programs (sets of synergies for Bernstein, 1967) and internal representations of the surrounding space and of the mechanical properties of their limbs.

- *Structuring of space*

Information from different sensory receptors during the action of subjects on their environment is used progressively to build a representation of the surrounding space which is structured by several frames of co-ordinates or reference frames (Paillard, 1991). Voluntary movements unroll in captured spaces (visual and manual captured spaces) which ensure the co-ordination of the egocentric space organised around postural referentials (position of the head and gaze in space, body axis) and the allocentric space of objects and places.

Goal directed movements are planned in an allocentric space defined by the task, for example the trajectory of the hand for a reaching movement (Ghez et al., 1991).

The execution of the movements can be explained as a progressive co-ordinate transformation of the spatial attributes of the target in visual space into information related to the action of muscles on articulations (Soechting and Flanders, 1992). The direction of the programmed movement is coded as a vector computed by the population of cortical cells from the visual position of the target and the initial position of the limb (Caminiti et al., 1991). The amplitude of the movement could be coded either as a scale factor (module of the vector) or by parallel coding of the end point of the movement.

- *Geometry and mechanical properties of the limb*

The simplest voluntary movement must account for the complex mechanical properties of the limb. The multi-jointed geometry of the limb implies that its stiffness, viscosity and inertia (which describe the dynamic relation between force and displacement) vary with its configuration (Lacquaniti, 1992). Accordingly, roboticians have highlighted the complexity of computations needed to transform an intended position into articular torques (known as the inverse dynamic problem).

Numerous neurophysiological studies have provided evidence that the motor command includes an anticipation of the perturbation that would arise from its own mechanical effects (Massion, 1992). This implies that the central nervous system must be endowed with an internal model of limb geometry and mechanics (Lacquaniti et al., 1992). Such representations are not conscious: when a person has planned a reaching movement towards an object, it is executed in a smooth, effortless manner which masks the great complexity of the dynamics of the arm. These representations are probably built in parallel with the body schema during the interaction with the environment; they are permanently updated to adapt to changing conditions. This adaptation is clearest in experiments carried out in micro-gravity conditions during space flights.

- *Trajectory formation*

The duration of aiming movements is prolonged when the target is small i.e. when the movement requires a higher degree of accuracy with a logarithmic relation known as Fitt's law (Fitt, 1954). Otherwise, the duration of a movement may be voluntarily scaled independent of its amplitude. Kinematic analysis has shown that the velocity profile is an invariant characteristic of flexion-extension movements of varied duration and amplitude. More generally, aiming movements executed in a plane (Abend et al., 1982) or in 3D space (Soechting and Flanders, 1992) are characterised by a rectilinear trajectory of the extremity of the limb and a bell-shaped velocity profile. When the trajectory is constrained by the task, as in drawing or writing movements, the tangential velocity of the movement is proportional to the radius of curvature of the trajectory (Viviani and Terzuolo, 1982).

These characteristics correspond to an optimisation or smoothing of the movement (Hogan & Flash 1987) but the mechanism of trajectory formation remains under discussion: it could be interpreted either as a succession of equilibrium points (Feldman, 1986) or as an emerging property of arm dynamics (Bullock & Grossberg, 1988).

Manipulative actions

Manipulation implies that subjects have acquired a representation of the physical properties of objects. This ability has been known for some time in the realm of developmental psychology (Piaget, 1936) and it is beginning to be explored with neurophysiological methods (see a review in Johansson and Cole, 1992). The internal representations of the properties of physical objects are demonstrated by the fact that motor commands involving objects are executed with anticipatory control mechanisms.

- *Examples of neurophysiological analysis*

Different experimental paradigms are currently being explored.

a- Grasping

A prehension movement includes two components (reaching and grasping) which reflect the output of two independent and temporally coupled motor programs driven by visuomotor mechanisms (Jeannerod, 1988). During the reaching movement, which is similar to an aiming movement, the hand is shaped as a function of the shape, size and orientation of the object. The kinematics of the transport and of the shaping of the hand reflect a precise co-ordination in order to close the finger around the object at the end of the reaching phase. The adaptation of these commands occurs partly in advance of the movement and thus implies a reliance on internal memory.

b- Precision grip

In lifting tasks with precision grip Johansson has shown (review in Johansson and Cole, 1992) that grip and load forces can be adjusted to the expected object's weight and surface friction in order to produce a smooth lift and a stable grasp. Object-related representations may be demonstrated with objects with a misleading aspect. If the object is lighter than expected, the programmed load force is too strong and there will be an excessive loading force inducing an overshoot (Johansson and Westling, 1988). Conversely, if the object is heavier than expected it will be lifted only after several loading force pulses. When people have no previous representations of the weight of an object they often adopt a "probing strategy": they progressively increment the loading force by a series of pulses and the object is lifted when the total force overcomes its weight. A similar strategy is also adopted by children during development (Forsberg et al., 1992). The representation of the object properties (weight, frictional constraints) is progressively updated by the repetition of lifts. The representation of the object's weight may be scaled to its size as demonstrated by Gordon et al. (1991). The task was to lift a series of objects of different volumes, corresponding to different proportional weights. If they could see the object, or perceive its size haptically, the subjects were able to adapt their efforts in advance to the expected weight. This suggests that human beings have an abstract representation of the density of objects.

c- Predictable impact forces

Anticipatory control is also evident in tasks involving predictable loading or unloading (Massion, 1992). In ball catching (Lacquaniti et al., 1992) or bimanual actions such as passing an object from one hand to the other (Dufossé et al., 1985), it was demonstrated that anticipatory actions were able to minimise the perturbation arising from the impact of the object. These actions are precisely timed and scaled to the amount of expected impact, suggesting that subjects have internalised the mechanics of the objects' free fall due to gravity (Newtonian mechanics).

- *Motor planning, serial and parallel commands*

Natural manipulation implies previous cognitive planning (for example one can catch a cup either by the handle with the precision grip or a bowl with the whole hand) depending on the required task and makes use of the representation of the expected properties of the object (Arbib, 1981). The execution of the motor plan involves both serial and parallel commands. The task of displacing an object includes a transport movement of the hand, controlled in parallel with the preparation for grasping the object (Jeannerod, 1988), followed by a sequence of different phases that can be considered as partial sub-goals: contact with the object, lifting of the object, stabilisation, replacement on the table, release from grasp (Johansson & Cole, 1992).

Proprioception and motor learning

The above results illustrate the importance of anticipatory mechanisms based on the internal representation of the control of manipulative actions. Currently, the main problem is to determine the mechanisms involved in the construction of representations during motor learning and development and correspondingly to specify the role of proprioceptive afferents.

- *Psychological theories of motor learning*

Many experimental studies on motor learning have concentrated on the acquisition of particular motor skills (sports for example) or to arbitrary gesture sequences. Following Schmidt (1975), motor learning involves a recall schema (to produce responses) and a recognition schema (to evaluate correctness) which are both modified during learning through a comparison of the expected with the actual feedback resulting from the movement (See Fig. 1, next page). Special focus is placed on the signals ("knowledge of the result") indicating that the aim of the movement has been achieved.

More recently, it has been hypothesised that the acquisition of co-ordination during both motor learning (Kelso et al., 1981) and development (Thelen, 1990) corresponds to dynamic equilibrium in a complex open system.

- *Neural basis of motor learning*

The importance of the cerebral cortex in the control of movement has long been recognised. Recent experiments in the behaviour of monkeys provide evidence of the importance of distributed cortical areas in dynamic aspects of motor control (Kalaska & Crammond, 1992). The motor cortex probably participates in anticipatory control mechanisms and motor learning as shown by functional imagery experiments in man (PET scan for example). In addition, the cerebellum is also probably involved in motor learning (Burnod and Dufossé, 1991). The architecture of the cerebellum cortex is such that it could be the seat of the coding of distributed representations and of adaptive comparisons between the expected and the actual feedback of the movement.

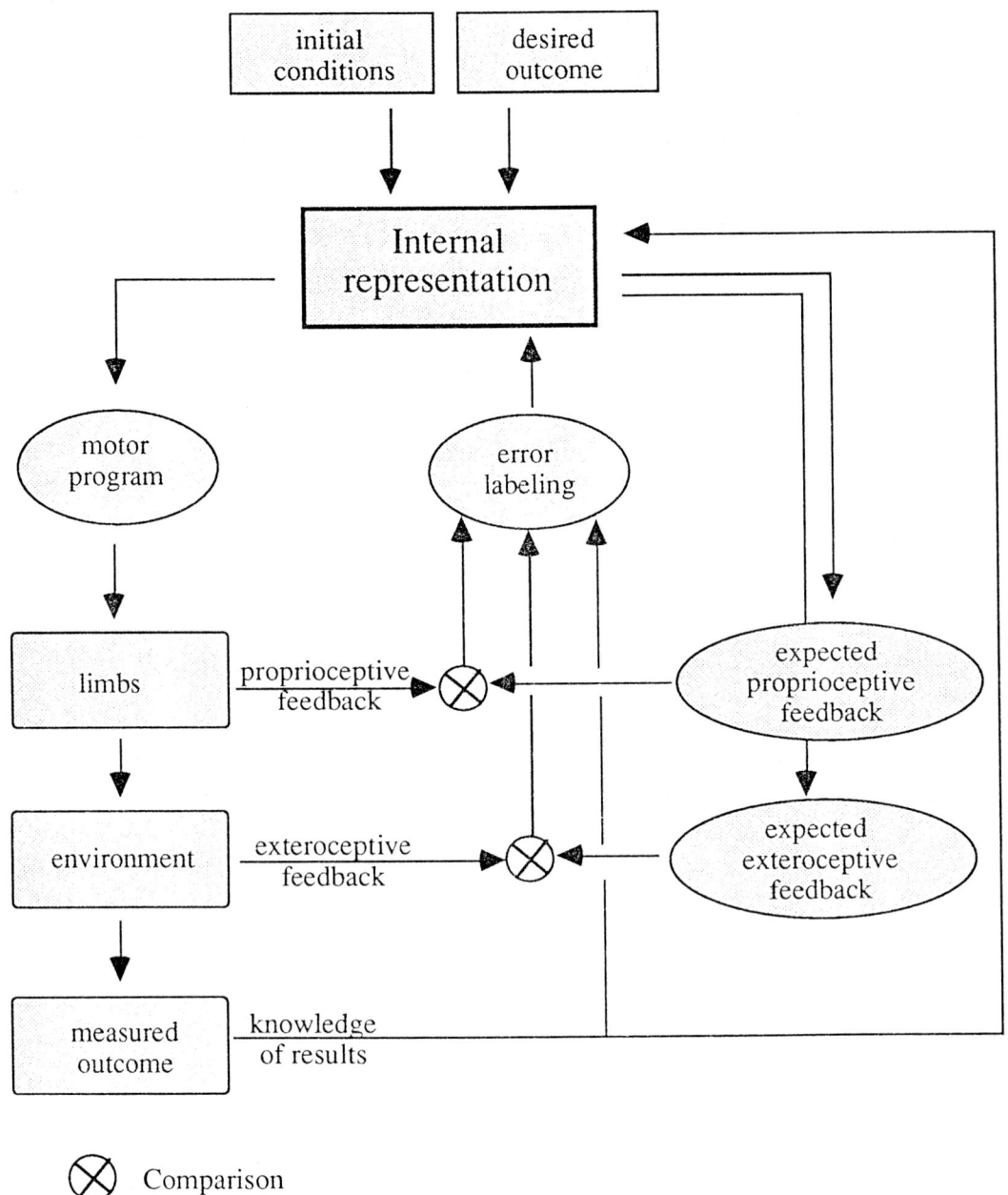

Fig. 1. Schema of the motor response in relation to events occurring within one gesture (adapted from Schmidt, 1975). Motor programs and representations are continuously updated through a comparison of the actual and expected sensory feedback.

• *Role of sensory afferents*

a- Afferents involved
Several kinds of sensory afferents are excited by self initiated movements. Proprioceptors (muscular and articular receptors) and some exteroceptors (such as cutaneous hand mechanoreceptors) are directly stimulated by movement. Visual information is obviously involved in visually guided behavior and it also signals, in keeping with vestibular information, any displacement of the head resulting from the movement. Auditory cues can also be used to guide a goal directed movement.

b- Feedback control processes
Sensory information concerning ongoing movement is not necessary for the completion of movement but improves its execution via a proper feedback control process (closed-loop on-line control). For example, pointing movements can still be executed if visual feed-back is altered by optical devices which hide the limb moving toward the target, but their accuracy is lower than under normal visual control (Beaubaton and Hay, 1986).

c- Feedforward control processes
Sensory information also has the role of amending future motor performance through a delayed adaptive loop. The adaptation or learning (see section on: Psychological theories of motor learning) results in a feedforward control which is able to anticipate the predictable constraints of motor execution on the basis of past experience. This means that information gathered during one particular movement is used to improve similar movements in the future. The computation leading to the motor error signal used in adaptive processes is still under discussion. The results obtained by Johansson et al. with precision grip (Johansson and Cole, 1992) suggest that part of the sensory-driven control could be discrete. An expected burst of activity in a particular group of afferents may signal that a subgoal of the movement has been completed (for example contact of the finger tips with the object or lift-off of the object) and may facilitate the unrolling of the movement sequence. Discrete sensory events can trigger responses to disturbances in a feed forward manner: a short (spontaneous or provoked) slip of the object induces a corrective rearangement of the grip co-ordination.

To conclude, the representation of the overall action probably includes continuous monitoring of both movement related signals (Paulignan et al., 1991) and discrete sensory events (Johansson and Cole, 1992) which are used to update the internal models.

INTERACTING WITH COMPUTERS

Description of sensori-motor interactions

• *Human-computer interface*

As described in detail by other authors in this seminar, the human-computer interface is a layer composed of interactive objects and it is relatively independent of the application and of human-computer dialog (Coutaz, 1990). In this context, an interaction means that all users' actions on the interface that modify the state of the computer application must produce a modification of the interface which is perceivable by users via one or more sensory modalities.

Conversely, the overall display of the objects of the interface must present the various actions that the users may choose as a function of the state of the application.

Recent advances in both the technology and ergonomy of interfaces have resulted in direct manipulation interfaces which now replace command languages and arbitrary interactions. Thus, interactions with computers are increasingly similar to interactions with objects in the real world and even emerge in virtual realities where data can be manipulated directly.

- *Place of gestures in man-machine interaction*

The place of gestures in human-computer interaction vary with the situations and the peripheral devices used.

a- Keyboards
Action on standard or chord keyboards needs complex gestures which impose prolonged motor learning. Movements by skilled typists have been studied extensively in relation to the layout of the keyboard and the semantic meaning of the keys. These data will not be presented here.

b- Direct manipulation
Due to the conception principle of the real-world metaphor, the use of direct manipulation interfaces is based on sensori-motor representations acquired during interactions with the real world. The present review is directed at the description of the devices and the modes of interactions within such direct manipulation interfaces.

c- Handwriting recognition
Another recent issue is the development of on-line handwriting recognition (Plamondon, 1991). Technological devices include the combinaison of a tablet digitizer and display on the same surface (as the recent Apple's "Newton"). Handwriting recognition poses similar problems to speech recognition (segmentation and pattern recognition of features, characters, words and semantic analysis). Algorithms used during the early stage of processing make use of shape recognition but also of the kinematic and dynamic characteristics of the trajectories of movements during writing (see section on:Trajectory formation).

- *Input devices used in direct manipulation interfaces*

In direct manipulation interfaces, data (for example a file representing a text) are represented by icons, usually displayed on a graphic video unit. Possible actions out are represented by the menus or by distinctive indices. The hierarchy of the actions is represented by unrolling lists of menu bars or by arrangements of nested or pop-up windows. The Graphic User Interface (GUI) may present a lot of information simultaneously to users who can actively explore the potentialities of the application or perform a goal-directed action. Physical gestures used to perform an action within the application are moulded by the nature of the input and output devices of the interface.

a- Touch sensitive screens
Touch sensitive screens are probably the most intuitive interfaces since the user acts directly on the icon represented on the screen.

The pointing gestures are identical to gestures directed on natural objects and, in particular, they unroll under normal visual control. The achievement of reaching is signalled by tactile information from the hand, by the vision of the fingertip above the icon and possibly by computer feedback (an auditory signal for example). The use of touch sensitive screens is highly dependant on vision.

b- Pressure sensitive tablets
In addition to tablet digitizers used for hand-writing recognition, pressure sensitive tablets with a lower spatial resolution can be used as input devices.
For example, the Concept Keyboard^{TM} offers 256 sensitive cells which can be grouped following the needs of the program and identified on an overlay. Pression on any of the group's cells induces the emission of a programmed string to the computer. With such interfaces, designation is identical to the designation movement in the natural world but the graphical display of the overlay cannot be modified as a function of the user's actions. With this kind of device, vision can be partly substituted by the haptic sense (tactile and proprioceptive information gathered during active exploration), particularly if the overlay includes raised marks (Hinton, Burger & al.in this volume).
The user probably constructs a representation of the location of the different commands in relation to the edges of the tablet and/or to his own postural frames of reference which can be used to guide further desired designation gestures.

c- Mouse and related devices.
Mouse and similar devices (trackballs) are now widespread in direct manipulation interfaces. The use of a computer mouse imposes a quite complex sensori-motor transformation. The user must learn the geometric spatial transformation between his gesture on the plane of the table and the displacement of the cursor on the screen and a multiplicative coefficient depending on the sensitivity of the mouse. Once this transformation is learned and generalised over the plane of the screen, any designation gestures can be performed in a feedforward manner, relying more on memory representation than on actual visual feedback.

Joysticks may also be used to drive a cursor on the screen. A joystick is a system of four perpendicularly arranged switches: the activation of one switch by an action on the stick induces a continuous displacement of the cursor in the corresponding direction. Similar effects can usually be obtained by iterative activations of the directional arrows of the keyboard.

Adapted switches can replace the joystick in the case of motor disability. Adapted switches are either standard but specially dressed switches (with long lever arms or big soft plastic "cushions" (Weiss, 1990)) or special switches designed to pick up biological signals such as puffs or electromyographical activity. Ocular movements in the four directions may be used to emulate four switches (Kaczmarek, 1992). If the motor disability is such that the user can act on only one switch the designation must include a scanning process directed by the program (scanning by lines and columns or by blocks).

TM Concept Keyboard is a trademark of Concept Keyboard Company ltd., United Kingdom.

d- Gaze direction.
It is possible with some optical methods to measure the direction of gaze independently of head movements. A hope for the future is to use gaze as an input device for people with massive motor disorders.

e- Data Glove ™
The metaphor of prehension within human computer interaction can be extended to 3D space with recent input devices in the form of clothing equipped with optical fibres that can sense the angular position of articulations. The data glove can recognise both the configuration of the hand (with optical fibres) and its 3D position and orientation (with an electromagnetic field device).

In the same way as the movement of a mouse drives the movement of a cursor on the screen, the movement of the hand clothed with the glove drives the movement of an "echo" on the screen (Fig. 2). The human computer interface may use different input signals: the position of the hand in reference to the work place, movements of the hand (translation movements, rotation of the wrist) or the configuration of the hand (i.e. the flexion-extension state of the fingers and thumb, plus the abduction of the thumb). Applications of the data glove and other 3D input devices have only just begun to be explored, for example data gloves are an essential component of virtual reality (see section on:Virtual reality) and may be used to enter complex gestural commands (see section on: Gestural commands).

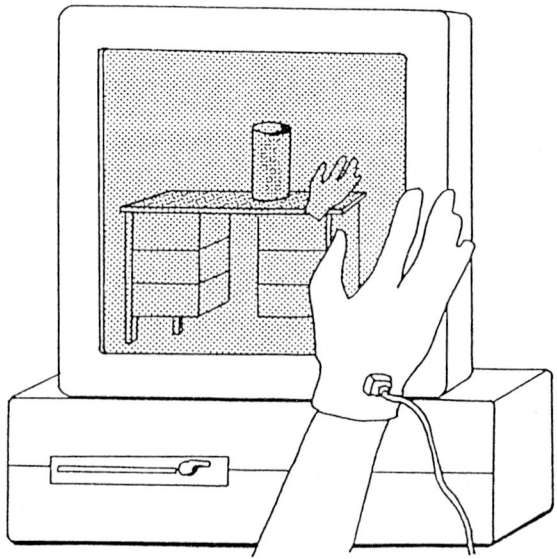

Fig. 2. Example of navigation in a 3D scene with the data glove. The configuration, position and orientation of the hand are used to pilot an "echo" of the glove through an abstract 3D representation (extension of the desk metaphor). Adapted from Bohm (1992)

™ Data Glove is a trademark of VPL Technologies ltd;, USA.

The concept of clothing devices has been extended to body suits which are mainly used to facilitate image synthesis in video applications.

• Virtual reality

Virtual realities (VR) are computer created three dimensional models combined with input and output devices that provide the most "natural" interactive situations.

The current state of virtual reality technology requires expensive computer power. Users perceive the model via a visual and auditory 3D display. The illusion of a 3D visual field is given by the simultaneous display of sophisticated 3D graphics on two little screens placed in front of each eye (with goggles or a helmet). In a similar way, real time calculation of audio signals presented to headphones may create the illusion that the sound comes from all around the user. The movements of the user are tracked by head position or orientation sensors, force plates beneath the user's seat, data gloves or body suits.

The principle of virtual reality is based on the fact that the 3D display is continuously modified by the users' movements, just as their perception of the real world would change as they move.

So, VR creates the illusion that the user is within an artificial environment. VR applications are often based on the metaphor of the "visit": navigation in the application may literally be an illusory locomotor activity.

VR has extensive potential applications for people with disabilities but these applications are currently limited by the cost of the equipment (Lanier, 1992). In particular, VR could provide a safe environment for learning and practising skills. Some applications of VR for people with disabilities are now being developed in several areas: assessment of function, assistive input technology for the mobility impaired, alternative communication devices (Greenleaf, 1992).

• Force displays

As evidenced above (see section on: Proprioception and motor learning), proprioceptive information is essential for motor control and learning. Accordingly, a current trend is to enhance direct manipulation interfaces with tactile or force feedback. For example, in a multimodal mouse (Akamatsu & Sato, 1991) the contact of the cursor with an icon is signalled by the rise of a small pin pressing the finger tip and the crossing of a window border is signalled by an increased resistance of the mouse's displacement due to an electromagnet. The multimodal mouse increases precision and reduces the duration of the pointing movement.

An input device with a built-in force feedback must both assure the measure of the subject's action (a displacement or a strain) and resist this action as a function of the properties of the simulated system (Cadoz, 1992). The most appealing applications of force displays are related to the prehension of virtual objects by the "echo" of the data glove in virtual reality. Force feedback has been used to signal the resistance to deformation of virtual objects as a function of their mechanical properties (Burdea et al., 1992).

Force displays are probably a key issue in rendering the direct manipulation of virtual objects more realistic. However, the full development of force interaction models must include the dynamics of the human arm under voluntary control which raises some complicated problems (see section on: Movement and representation). Advances in this field will probably parallel advances in robotics, particularly in the design of telemanipulation systems.

Implications of sensori-motor representations for direct manipulation interfaces

• *Screen layout and representation*

Whatever the device employed to drive the cursor, active exploration probably allows the user to build a representation of the location of the constant icons representing the commands on the screen (menu bars). A particular command corresponds to a sequence of actions that can be memorised and parametrised as a function of the initial location of the cursor.

This learning is facilitated by the actual standardisation of graphical interfaces. For example, to activate the function "Save File", the user must know the sequence:
- displace the cursor to the upper left corner of the screen
- select the menu "FILES"
- drag the cursor downwards N steps
- select the option "Save File".

Visual feedback signalling the unrolling of the menu bars may be used more to synchronise the gestures and control the sequential execution of the commands than to directly guide the gestures.

• *3D layout.*

Screen layout could be generalised to 3D interfaces or virtual reality. Actions in the virtual world would be directed by the sensori-motor representation acquired during active exploration. This field is still largely experimental and the human factors intervening in 3D interactions with computer are only beginning to be explored.

Despite the fact that virtual reality currently relies mainly on graphic 3D displays, future applications will probably be encouraging for people with reduced visual function. The nested windows of the actual GUI are in fact 3D constructions which are almost inaccessible to the blind. The development of 3D sound and force displays could probably give access to 3D computer layouts for the blind since they would be available directly by manipulation. Indeed, the haptic sense may be accurately substituted for vision for active exploration and recognition in blind as in blindfolded people (Hatwell, 1986).

• *Gestural commands*

In addition to direct manipulation of data, mouse type devices or data gloves can be used to generate gestural commands. The same intermediary steps exist between the metaphorically "natural" pointing movements or manipulation of virtual objects and gestural commands with a particular semantic meaning.

Gestures usually accompany speech in natural human communication and ensure a particular semantic signification. Ekman and Friesen (1972) distinguish "emblems" (for example the gesture to say "good-bye") and "illustrators" that supplement meaning by pointing, emphasising, demarcating etc...(for example "look at this book"). Gestural communication may substitute for speech when the acoustic mode cannot be used, for example the sign language used by deaf people or the codes used in particular environments (scubadiving etc...).

Both emblematic and illustrative gestural commands can be used in human computer communication (Morrel-Samuels, 1990). Recent developments are based on the semantic signification of gestures recorded in 2D with a mouse or a digitising tablet (Rubine, 1991) or in 3D with a data glove (Braffort, 1991). For example, in one particular toolkit, a circular gesture around a set of icons is used to select data; the prolongation of the gesture indicates a displacement; a stroke across the icon is used to delete the data (Kurtenbach and Buxton, 1991).

Gestural commands similar to proofreadering marks may also be used for text editing in association or not with handwriting recognition.

The conventional mark "√" is both an emblem of the verb "INSERT" and an illustrator for the place where to insert (Morrel-Samuels, 1990). With the data glove a particular movement may signal an action (move forward) and the configuration of the hand (3 fingers extended) a parameter of the action (move 3 pages) (Braffort, 1991).

Observation of movements and ergonomic analysis

The purpose of direct manipulation interfaces is to provide the most "natural" kinds of information. However, interaction with computers implies bridging the gap between the space of commands where the action is performed and the space of control where the result of the action is displayed. The user has to learn the sensorimotor transformation imposed by the input-output arrangement of the interface. This learning process is usually short and easy with recent interfaces but may be much more difficult for people with sensory and/or motor disabilities. So, the observation of movements during learning may provide a useful method of analysis of sensori-motor problems confronted during human-computer interactions.

- *Trajectory recording*

As seen above (see section on: Trajectory formation), the trajectory of a goal directed movement in the natural world is roughly linear with a bell-shaped velocity profile. This kinematic analysis shows an optimisation of the movement and suggests that the person has an accurate representation of the movement to be carried out and of its sensory consequences. These considerations can be extended to 2D gestures in human computer interactions (Roby-Brami, 1992). When using a mouse, expert subjects make linear pointing movements with bell-shaped velocity profiles. In comparison, the first pointing movements made by novices are highly variable (Fig. 3). After an initial learning period (about 10 trials), novices learn to anticipate the consequences of their actions on the mouse on the cursor movements. However, novices' movements remain more variable and less accurate than those of expert users.

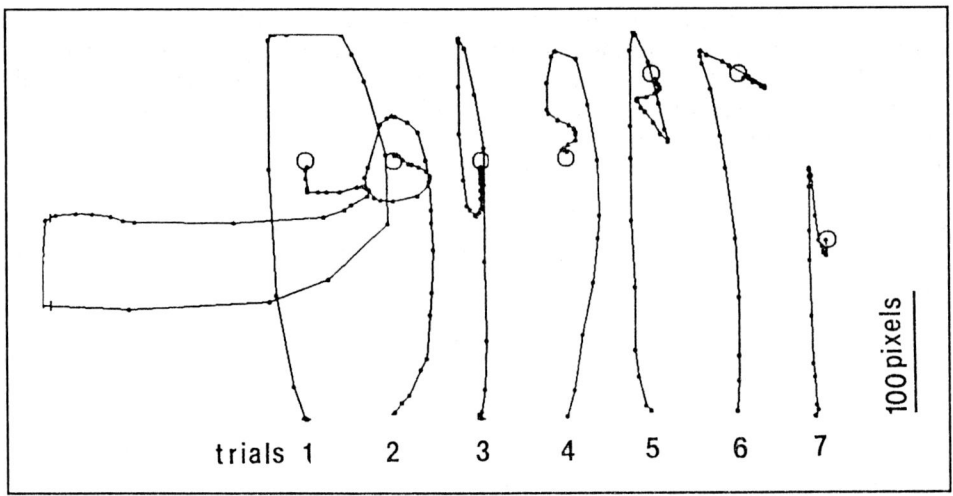

Fig 3. Example of mouse cursor trajectories recorded during the firsts trials by a novice user. The goal of the movement was to position the cursor on the target (wide circle). The position of the cursor was sampled at 18.9 Hz (each small circle represents one sample).

Kinematics methods could be useful in improving learning conditions for people with sensori-motor disabilities. First, the on-line display of the trajectory characteristics or of added sensory feedback may facilitate learning (see section on: Role of sensory afferents). Second, analysis of the trajectory by the ergonomist or therapist may highlight particular problems. Third, in the near future, kinematic data could be used to transfer a part of the learning process to some adaptive computation inserted within the interface.

- *Hand as a tool*

The human hand is a powerful tool both in the acquisition of information about the environment and in the transformation of this environment. The observation of hand movements and configurations may shed light on the psycho-physiological mechanisms involved during a manipulative task (review in Hatwell 1986). Motor strategies vary as a function of the haptic characteristics of the object (softess, texture, weight.). Similarly, the shaping of the hand varies according to the intended action on the environment. The demonstration of anticipatory mechanisms during manipulative tasks (see section on: Manipulative actions) predicts that the observation of the configuration reflects subjects' representations of the task. So, the recording of hand shape with a data glove or quantitative video analysis could be a valuable method of investigating human-computer interactions.

CONCLUSION

Direct manipulation interfaces represent a growing trend in methods of interactions with computers. This evolution is due to the increasing attention given to human factors. As claimed by Lanier "the goal is to see how you can use technology and mold it to a person instead of asking a person to come to the technology". The increasing individualisation of the interfaces follows from this trend and this perspective represents a real hope for people with a sensory-motor disability.

The development of semantically meaningful gestural commands is promising for visually impaired people. Direct manipulation commands in human-computer interfaces are mostly visually guided gestures but also appeal to the other sensory systems such as audition or the haptic sense. So, gestures could be an accessible communication mode for visually impaired people. The problem for visually impaired users is the necessity to learn the sensori-motor actions in order to obtain a desired command. This evidence underlines the interest of further theoretical studies on sensori-motor learning processes in order to specify adaptation mechanisms and particularly the effects of sensory messages and "error signals" produced by an action. In the future, one can imagine that a part of the learning process could be delegated to an "intelligent" layer of the interface including formal neural nets. In addition, the development of multimodality will probably increase the possibilities of sensory feedback and thus improve the methods of interaction particularly during the learning period.

REFERENCES

Abend W., Bizzi E. & Morasso (1982), Human arm trajectory formation,, *Brain 105*, p.331-348.

Akamatsu M. & Sato S. (1991), Development of Multi-Modal integrative mouse. Mouse type interface device with tactile and force display, *7th Human Interface Symposium*, Kyoto, 1991.

Arbib M.A. (1981), Perceptual structures and distributed motor control, *Handbook of Physiology, Vol 2*, Motor control, VB Brook éditeur, American physiological society, Bethesda, p 1449-1480.

Beaubaton D. & Hay L. (1986), Contribution of visual information to feedforward and feedback processes in rapid pointing movements, *Human Movement Science*, 5, p.19-34.

Bernstein M. (1967), *Co-ordination and regulation of movements*, New York: Pergamon Press.

Bohm(1992), GIVEN: An interface toolkit for 3D interaction, In *Interface to real and virtual worlds, EC2, Informatique 92*, Montpellier.

Braffort A. (1992), Definition d'un modèle d'interaction pour gant numérique, *Mémoire de DEA, Université Paris XI*, LIMSI.

Bullock D. & Grossberg S. (1988), Neural dynamics of planned arm movements: emergent invariants and speed acuracy properties during trajectory formation, *Psychological Reviews 95*, p.49-90.

Burdea G., Roskos E., Silver D., Thibaud F. & Wolpov R. (1992), A distributed virtual environment with dextrous force feedback, In *Interface to real and virtual worlds, EC2, Informatique 92*, Montpellier, p.255-265.

Burnod Y. (1989), *An adaptive neural network, the cerebral cortex*, Masson, Paris.

Burnod Y. & Dufossé M., *A model for the cooperation between cerebral cortex and cerebellar cortex in movement learning*, In Brain and space, Paillard ed., Oxford Science publications, p 446-458.

Burnod Y., Grandguillaume P., Otto I., Ferraina S., Johnson P.B. & Caminiti R. (1992), Visuomotor transformations underlying Arm Movements toward Visual targets: A Neural Network Model of Cerebral Cortical Operations, *Journal of Neuroscience, 12*, p.1435-1453.

Cadoz C. (1992), Interface de communication instrumentale : clavier retroactif modulaire , In *Interface to real and virtual worlds, EC2, Informatique 92*, Montpellier, p.43-47.

Caminiti R., Johnson P.B., Galli C., Ferraina S. & Burnod Y. (1991), Making arm movements within different parts of space: The premotor and motor cortical representation of a co-ordinate system for reaching to visual targets, *J. Neurosci. 11*, p.1182-1197.

Coutaz J. (1990), *Interfaces homme-ordinateur, conception et réalisation*, Paris: Dunod informatique, Bordas.

Dufossé M., Hugon M. & Massion J. (1985), *Postural forearm changes induced by predictable in time or voluntary triggered unloading in man*, Exp. Br. Res. 60, p.330-334.

Ekman P. & Friesen W. (1972), Hand movements, *J. of communication*, 22, p. 353-374.

Feldman A.G. (1986), Once more on the equilibrium point hypothesis (lambda model) for motor control, *J. Motor Behavior 18*, p.17-54.

Forssberg H., Kinoshita H., Eliasson A.C., Johansson R.S., Westling G. & Gordon A.M. (1992), *Development of human precision grip II: Anticipatory control of isometric forces targeted for objects's weight*, Exp. Br. Res. 90, p.393-398.

Ghez C., Hening W. & Gordon J. (1991), Organisation of voluntary movements, *Current Opinion in Neurobiology*, 1, p.664-671.

Gordon A.M., Forssberg H., Johansson R.S. & Westling G. (1991), *Integration of sensory information during the programming of precision grip : comments on the contribution of size cues*, Exp. Br. Res. 85, p.226-229.

Hatwell Y. (1986), *Toucher l'espace*, Presses Universitaires de Lille.

Hogan N. & Flash T. (1987), Moving gracefully: quantitative theories of motor co-ordination, *Trends in Neurosciences, 10*, p.170- 174.

Jeannerod M. (1988), *The neural and behavioural organisation of goal-directed movements*, Oxford, Clarendon Press.

Johansson R.S. & Cole K.J. (1992), Sensory-motor co-ordination during grasping and manipulative actions, *Current Opinion in Neurobiology, 2,*, p.815-823.

Johansson R.S. & Westling G. (1988), *Co-ordinated isometric muscle commands adequately and erroneously programmed for the weight during lifting task with precision grip*, Exp. Br. Res. 71, p.59-71.

Kalaska J.F. & Crammond D.J. (1992), Cerebral cortical mechanisms of reaching movements, *Science, 255*, p.1517-1523.

Kaczmarek R. (1992), Commande oculaire pour l'aide à la communication et au contrôle de l'environnement par l'handicapé moteur, *Motricité cérébrale 13*, p.24-30.

Kelso J.A.S., Holt K.G., Rubin P. & Kugler P.N. (1981), Patterns of human interlimb co-ordination emerge from the preperties of non-linear, limit cycle oscillatory processes: theory and data, *J. Motor behavior, 13*, p.226-261.

Kurtenbach G. & Buxton B. (1991), GEDIT : a test bed for editing by continuous gestures, *SIGCHI Bulletin*, April 1991, p.22-26.

Lacquaniti F., Borghese N.A. & Carrozzo M. (1992), *Co-ordinate transformations in the control of limb stiffness*, Exp. Br. Res. Series 22, p.17-25.

Lanier J. (1992), Virtual reality and persons with disabilities, *Proceedings of the 7th annual international conference "Technology and persons with disabilities"*, Los Angeles, p.2-6.

Massion J. (1992), Movement, posture and equilibrium: interaction and co-ordination, In progress in *Neurobiology, Vol 38*, p35-56.

Morrel-Samuels P. (1990), Clarifying the distinction between lexical and gestural commands, *Int. J. Man-machine Studies, 32*, p.581-590.

Newell C. (1992), Theme issue on dynamical approaches to motor skill acquisition, *J. Motor Behavior, 24, 1*.

Paulignan Y., Jeannerod M., Mackenzie C. & Marteniuk R. (1991), *Selective perturbation of visual input during prehension movements*, 2, The effects of changing object size, Exp. Br. Res. 87, p.407-420.

Paillard J. (1991), Motor and representational framing of space, In *Brain and space, Paillard ed.*, Oxford Science publications, p 163-182.

Piaget J. (1936), *La naissance de l'intelligence chez l'enfant*, Neuchâtel, Delachaux et Niestlé.

Plamondon R. (1991), Steps toward the design of an electronic pen-pad, In *Interface to real and virtual worlds, EC2, Informatique 92*, Montpellier, p.201-214.

Roby-Brami A. (1992), gesturPointing es in man-machine interface, Analysis of the mouse cursor trajectory, *Proceedings of the 14th annual international conference of the IEEE-EMBS*, Paris, 4, p.1656-1657.

Rumelhart D.E. & Mc Clelland J.L. (1986), *Parallel distributed processing, Explorations in the microstructure of cognition*, *Vol 1* Foundations., MIT press, Cambridge, Massachusetts.

Schmidt R.A. (1975), A schema theory of discrete motor skill learning, *Psychological reviews, 82*, p.225-260.

Soechting J.F. & Flanders M. (1992), Moving in three dimensional space : frames of reference, vectors and co-ordinate systems, *Ann. Rev. Neurosci. 15*, p.167-191.

Thelen E . (1990), Coupling perception and action in the development of skill : a dynamic approach, In *Sensori-motor organisations and development in infancy and early childhood*, Bloch H et Berthental BI éditeurs, Kluwer academic publishers, The Netherlands, p.39-56.

Viviani P. & Terzuolo C. (1982), Trajectory determines movement dynamics, *Neuroscience, 7*, p.431-437.

Von Hofsten C. (1991), Structuring of early reaching movements: a longitudinal study, J. *Motor Behavior, 23*, p.280-292.

Weiss P.L. (1990), Mechanical characteristics of microswitches adapted for the physically handicapped, *J. Biomed. Eng. 12*, p.398-402.

Ziegler J.E. & Fehnrich K.P. (1990), Direct manipulation, In *Handbook of human computer interaction*, Helander M editeur, North Holland, Amsterdam, p.123-133.

Résumé

La manipulation d'objets dans le monde réél implique que la personne qui agit ait acquis les représentations sensori-motrices nécessaires à son action sur l'environnement. Ce texte présente une revue de travaux en psychophysiologie montrant que les gestes dirigés vers un but sont réalisés de façon anticipatrice. Les mécanismes proposés pour expliquer l'apprentissage sensori-moteur sont exposés. Les interactions sensori-motrices qui se produisent dans les interfaces homme-ordinateur sont analysées à la lumière de ces données. Enfin est abordé le problème de la conception d'interfaces adaptées pour les personnes présentant une déficience sensorielle ou motrice.

The design of interactive auditory learning tools

Dominique Burger, Christian Mazurier[1], Serge Cesarano[1] and Jack Sagot[1]

INSERM U 88, Groupe CREARE, 91, boulevard de l'Hôpital, 75013 Paris, France, et [1] CNEFEI, 58-60, avenue des Landes, 92150 Suresnes, France

ABSTRACT

Sounds are an important part of our environment that contribute to our understanding of the surrounding world. From early childhood on, sounds and the auditory channel play an important role in the learning process. The purpose of this paper is to discuss how technology may help create interactive auditory material that can be used to teach blind children. First, the power of paper-based materials for education is recalled. Then, substitution materials used to teach the visually impaired are presented. Finally, various computer systems developed and experimented in schools by the authors are presented in order to illustrate how multimodal interaction techniques allow manipulation and transformation of auditory objects located in two-dimensional space. This supports the argument that technology might soon bring about metaphorical environments which may be as useful for the blind as images are for sighted people.

THE USE OF IMAGES IN EDUCATION

Images on paper play a central role in the educational process of sighted children, mainly because images provide useful substitutes for real objects. Both mental and physical operations can be carried out on images in a way similar to that in reality. Pictures give children many opportunities to explore, identify, analyse, classify, or verbalise about things or scenes. Pencils, scissors, paste and other low cost tools allow them to transform or build up images.

In fact, images often appear to be even more useful than real objects because they are not bulky and are inexpensive, manageable, easy to copy and circulate. Moreover, their stability over time frees children from time constraints during training.

In addition, images constitute an intermediate stage between the real world and the world of ideas, concepts and symbols. Things have to be idealised in order to be put onto a sheet of paper. For instance, some features have to be removed, in particular three-dimensionality and movement, while some significant characteristics are emphasised. Images can be devised and designed according to specific pedagogical needs.

For instance, abstractions such as geometric shapes or collections that are unlikely to be found in the classroom can be represented. Textual comments can also be mixed with the images. Last but not least, in our modern society, images constitute common and consensual vehicles for either conceptual or emotional communication with which almost everyone feels at ease and finds useful in many situations.

Obviously paper-based activities rely on the capacity of vision to grasp images in their entirety extremely rapidly, and at the same time to identify significant patterns and to understand spatial and logical relationships between them. The visual system has a wide range of sophisticated processing mechanisms involved in the extraction of such complex tasks, including filtering, pattern recognition and parallel processing.

Psychologists would summarise by saying that images constitute suitable environments in which children can construct, verify and reinforce forms of thinking through concrete experience. As a result, paper-based materials are widespread and used for educational purposes by both teachers and parents.

In contrast, educational materials available for visually handicapped children are poor, scarce and expensive. Once blind children have learned to read and count, it becomes extremely difficult to find appropriate books to teach them about the world and to access culture. But even before then, blind children suffer from a lack of rich educational or recreational environments. This situation has often been hypothesised by psychologists to be one of the causal factors in the delayed development often observed in cognitive skills such as classification, abstract reasoning or spatial ability (Fraiberg, 1977; Schneekloth, 1989; see also Hatwell in this volume).

MATERIALS AVAILABLE FOR TEACHING BLIND CHILDREN

Therefore, educators have developed materials intended to fulfil the same general objectives as traditional teaching materials and to match the special needs of visually handicapped children. The following section briefly describes frequently used materials and emphasises their limitations in comparison with visual material.

Scale models of objects

Scale models of objects are often used by educators to allow children to perceive spatial features in order to explain about volumes and the relationships between functional parts. For instance, blind children are thus able to experience an elephant, its trunk, and its size compared with that of a cat, an experience that is not accessible to them through seeing or touching a real elephant. Such materials can be cheap, off-the-shelf products, but they are also sometimes especially designed and created. Their manipulation needs space. Their transformation is neither easy nor encouraged.

Manipulatives

Many educational kits have been designed to encourage active attitudes in visually impaired children and to develop hand and finger co-ordination, dexterity, tactile discrimination and, last but not least, abstract thinking. They generally include objects, cubes, rods, shapes and laces, whose colour and texture have been devised to be clearly perceivable. Their design often involves clever ideas intended to make discovery and manipulation attractive and enjoyable. In some cases, auditory features are added to reinforce perception and fun. Since they are almost always especially designed for the blind, and are frequently one-purpose oriented, such kits often appear to be rather expensive.

Tactile diagrams

Tactile diagrams are widely used in the education of the blind. Various techniques are used to produce raised images including embossing, thermoforming and photocopiers using special inks that swell when heated. Thermoforming is very widespread since tactile diagrams which are generally obtained by hand can be reproduced very simply from an initial matrix with a photocopy-like method.

Objects in this form are usually represented in 2-D static space, so tactile images have some similarities with printed ones. Nevertheless, it must be emphasised that their perception is quite different. Thus, conversion of visual information into a tactile form is a specific job that has to take into account strict rules in order to convey information efficiently (see Hinton in this volume).

Another point is that transformation of tactile information by the students themselves is not easy, so that such materials are generally proposed as an illustration rather than intended to be tinkered with.

One major difficulty with tactile diagrams concerns their annotation in braille. As stated by Hinton (1991): "Because of the unavoidable space which the braille script takes up it comes to dominate what is on the page, in the mind of the designer if not overtly in the finished product". One solution is to remove braille annotations from the illustration and to provide the user with alphanumeric keys to clarify the relationships between the tactile diagrams and captions. This approach involves unavoidable disruptions during the reading process.

Audio-tactile diagrams

The NOMAD system has been developed in an attempt to overcome this difficulty (Parkes, 1991). The whole system consists of a computer, a speech synthesiser and a sensitive tablet. When tactile diagrams are set up on the tablet, software allows messages to be attached to some locations of the diagram and to vocalise them on request by pressing the corresponding location. So prepared tactile diagrams are called audio-tactiles. They prove to be a powerful illustration technique in many fields, such as geography, biology or technology (see Hinton in this volume). Despite the fact that they embed sound, audio-tactiles are mainly touch-based materials.

Tape-recorded materials

Cassettes provide a low-cost vehicle for auditory material. They can contain verbal or non-verbal material and can be accessed by a standard tape-recorder . Many activities can be based on listening, including speech and language, memory, counting, music or motor activities. Audio-materials can offer a wide variety of life-like contents. Therefore they provide opportunities for entertaining and emotionally rich activities. But auditory-based activities need continuous and sustained attention. This severely limits the duration of training sessions especially within groups. The fact that reading is mainly sequential is also a limiting factor.

THE POTENTIAL OF INTERACTIVE AUDITORY ENVIRONMENTS

Computers create new conditions for both sound production and the possible use of sound-based materials for education. Sounds can be either sampled or reproduced with high fidelity. High quality musical sounds can be computed and produced in real time so that the storage of long pieces of music is no longer a problem. Spoken messages can also be obtained from text in real time with a pretty high level of intelligibility.

These facilities are now available on most personal computer systems thanks to specific peripherals. The trend observed in the evolution of so-called multimedia computers is to embed some of these possibilities in basic computer set-ups, and to provide full compatibility with mass-production devices such as CD-Audio readers, as well as sound creating and editing software. The cost of all these facilities is falling rapidly.

But, beyond this, probably the most radical changes are to be expected from progress made in human-computer interactions techniques. Over the last few years, we have become convinced that sound technology and the great variety of new peripherals constitute a great potential for the development of learning tools for the blind. Thus, a great deal of our research effort has been concentrated on the design and implementation of technological environments in which blind children are given the possibility of manipulating sounds in the same way as they would with pieces of lego.

Three different projects will now be described. The PolySon and SoundBench projects were completed some time ago. They engendered the current TactiSon project which has important implications for the topics discussed in this conference. Thus, Polyson and Soundbench will be described briefly, whereas full details will be given about TactiSon.

PolySon

PolySon is an autonomous microprocessor-based device that has been developed and used for some years in classrooms with visually-impaired students whose ages range from about 5 to 10 years (Burger et al, 1987; Burger et al., 1990). It provides facilities for building sound sequences from basic fragments, i.e. musical tones, noises and spoken words.

Sounds are characterised by four parameters 1) speed, 2) intensity, 3) pitch and 4) timbre which can be varied independently. Commands are sent to Polyson through an input device which can be either:
- an optical reader which is able to recognise punched cards receiving up to 7 perforations, thus coding up to 128 different words.
- a bar-code reader allowing the use of bar-coded sheets containing either basic commands or macro-commands.

Commands have the general form: *Command + Numerical Parameter*. Thus children have to learn a simple but specific language. The nature of the input devices means that teachers have considerable freedom in the choice of appropriate words or symbols to name commands. Labelling can be in either large print or braille.

Many learning situations were designed and tested by or with teachers, covering sound awareness, logic tasks, metalinguistic training and programming activities.

Soundbench

The Soundbench project was developed to accomplish similar objectives to PolySon. However, the technology and the interface system on which they are based are quite different since a Macintosh™ computer is used. MacRecorder™ is used to sample, prepare and produce sounds. A HyperCard™ stack is used to create an auditory and graphical user interface that can be operated by either a mouse or a touch screen device. Characteristic sounds are used to reinforce the perception of events occurring on the screen, for instance when the mouse pointer encounters an object or when a command is being executed (Fig. 1). The basic sounds intended to be used for auditory sequence construction are hierarchically organised, stored within boxes, that are to be found in cupboards. Limited experimentation was carried out with two 11 to 13 year-old totally blind students that led to encouraging conclusions especially concerning the use of spatialized interaction modes.

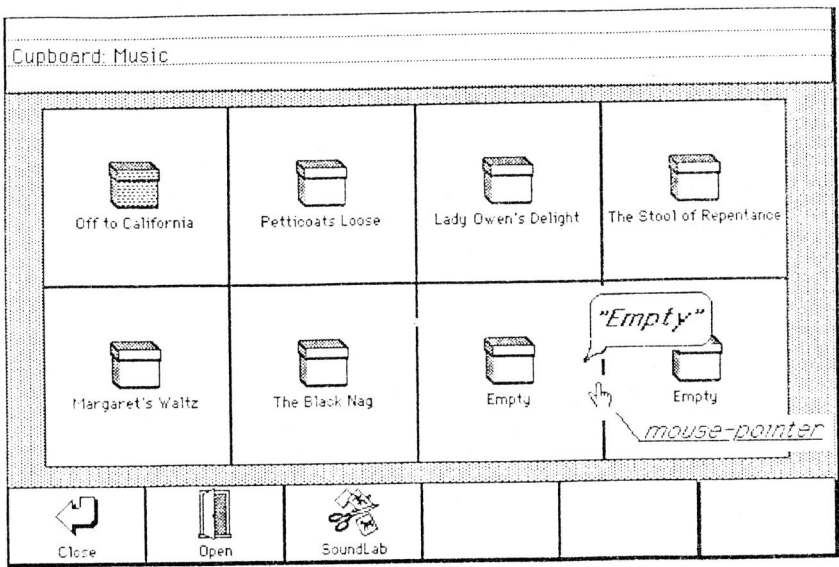

Fig. 1 shows a typical SoundBench screen The utterance of the message "Empty" occurs when the mouse enters the corresponding area.

Beyond these differences in the design of the interface system, it should be emphasised that both approaches are mainly command-mediated, which means that students interact with a computer to act on remote things. (Fig. 2a) Even with the sophistication of a GUI-like interface that was made possible by HyperCard, this approach involves indirect manipulation of the objects on which the actions are performed.

Both the generalisation of direct manipulation in the human-computer interaction systems and its particular adequation to the question of helping children to construct efficient representations of the world has resulted in us concentrating on bridging the gap between users and manipulated sounds. This has led to the current project which will be described and discussed in detail in the following sections.

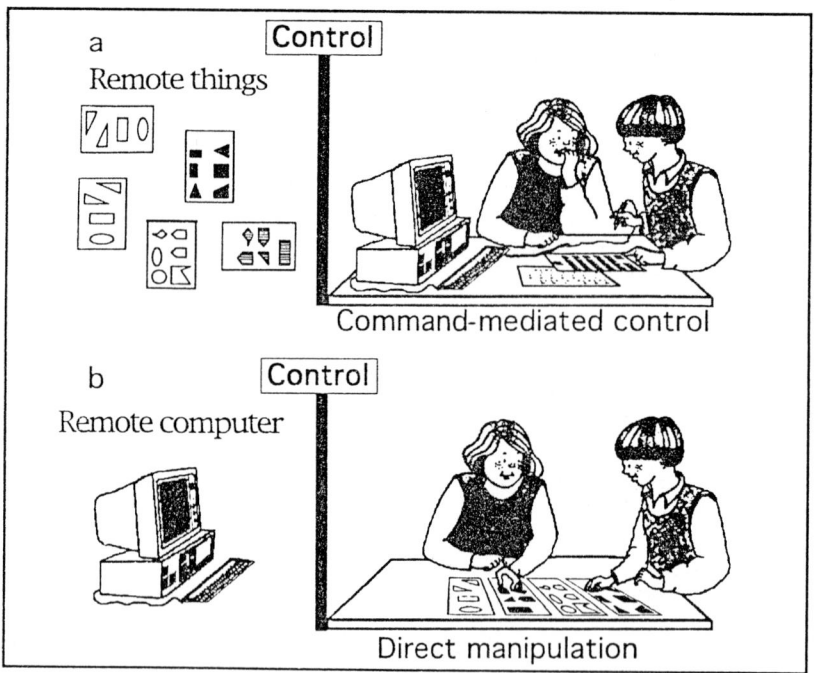

*Fig. 2 illustrates the difference between command-mediated, hence **indirect**, and **direct** manipulations in human-computer interactions.*

TACTISON

General purpose

In order to give users the illusion of manipulable objects, interface systems have to give the impression of a physical presence (Fig 2b). In a GUI, this generally means object-like images moving within the 2-D space of the screen. For people who cannot see the screen properly, the interface has to address sensory modalities other than vision. In fact, both haptic and auditory perception have to be involved to give a good illusion.

This was the major concern in Tactison and the reason why it inherited its central technique from Nomad, i.e. a two-dimensional sensor and sound production features. The principle of manipulating sounds like Lego pieces was retained from Polyson and Soundbench.

A useful metaphor

A metaphor can be used to understand Tactison. Imagine a tray containing objects which you cannot see because they are covered by a sheet of paper or cardboard, an overlay (Fig. 3). You can however hear them since they emit a sound as soon as they are touched. Obviously, your interest and attention will not focus on the overlay itself but on the objects hidden underneath, in particular when you discover that they produce different sounds depending on the way you touch them, on whether you click, double-click or press. You can also move, cut and copy them. Overlays are not however a trifling matter since they carry raised marks that can help locate, identify and retrieve objects and thus contribute to the understanding of the overall organisation. Thus, the design of their tactile appearance has to be considered with care. Some overlays are divided into areas, like windows on a screen. In fact these areas can be understood as outlining boxes on the tray in which the objects are or can be arranged. Boxes represent another type of objects that can also utter messages when the finger clicks, double-clicks or presses them. But boxes are stuck to the back of the tray. They can therefore not be moved.

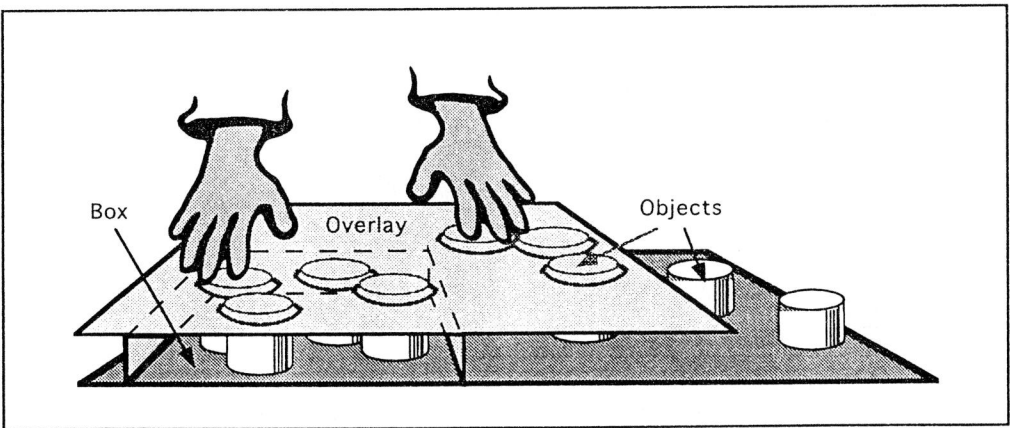

Fig. 3 illustrates the TactiSon metaphor

Such a metaphor may help to create a representation of the system using intuitive knowledge and concepts in a concrete domain with which users are familiar. It can also provide guidelines for teaching strategies or for vocabulary. Obviously, as with all metaphors, it will never fully match the characteristics and functions of the computer systems. Finally, such a metaphor seems to be rather consistent with everyday experiences of the blind who perceive objects by audition, reaching, manipulation and palpation.

Hardware implementation

Various considerations were taken into account in the choice of technologies. Cost, availability, and compatibility played an essential role. This led to a configuration based on a MS-DOS 286 (or higher) computer with at least 20Mo hard disk memory.

A Concept Keyboard ™ is used as sensitive input. This device has a 21x29.7 cm, A4-format and counts 256 active contacts whose lay-out is organised in 16-contact lines and 16-contact columns.

Sounds are produced by either a PSOLA ™ French speaking text-to-speech synthesiser or a TMPI ™ sampler based on the ADPCM compression technique.

Commands

A general principle in the design of human-computer interfaces is to reduce the number of actions executed by users and the number of concepts they must remember (Keiras & Bovair, 1984). As a matter of fact, only a few basic operations can provide many possible manipulations. The basic operative concepts were: reading, page turning, marking, cutting, moving and copying. Each can apply to various objects, in various situations.

A **read** command makes it possible to get information about the contents of a line, the contents of a column, the contents of a box and all the contents on the tray
A **turn page** command allows users to change exercise by loading the contents of another tray
A **mark** command is necessary in order to make an object special or noticeable
A **cut** command removes an object from the tray
A **move** command changes the position of an object on the tray
A **copy** command creates a clone of an existing object in a specified position on the tray

Design considerations

Tactile overlays

Some empirical rules of tactile design were followed (Fig. 4):

- very simple shapes for both abstract and figurative items,
- tactile hints and guidance
- symmetrical shapes as often as possible in order to make the pattern recognition process independent of the direction of finger exploration

Nevertheless, overlays were frequently revised after use by the students (Fig. 4c, 4d).

[TM] Concept Keyboard is a trademark of Concept Keyboard Ltd, United Kingdom
PSOLA is a trademark of Elan-Informatique, France
TMPI is a trademark of TechniMusique, France

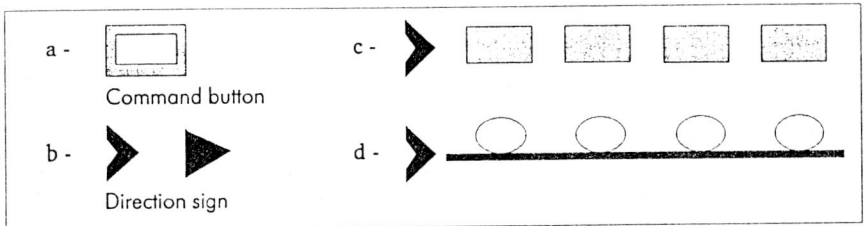

Fig. 4 shows some tactile patterns that were tested with children. Fig.4c shows a design which clearly evoked a line of objects when perceived by the eye. It had to be modified to make it clearly perceived as a line by touch (Fig. 4).

Lay-out (Fig. 5)

• Objects are always presented in the central of the overlay,
• Commands are presented at the periphery.
• If possible, things are presented in rows and columns in order to facilitate exploration. Once readers have understood this principle, they can guess the general organisation from only partial exploration. This can compensate for the loss of global perception. Such a regular arrangement also facilitates item retrieval.

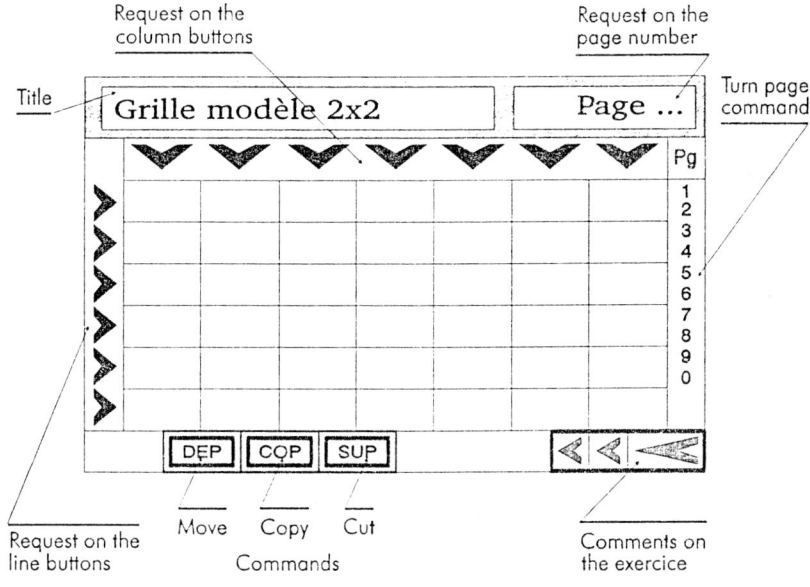

Fig. 5 shows the general lay-out that was adopted for the design of overlays.

105

Actions

As mentioned above, three types of physical actions can be carried out on the surface of an overlay, namely click, double-click and press. Each is precisely defined in time as shown in Fig. 6

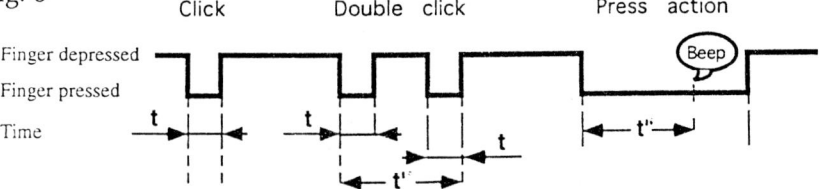

Fig. 6 illustrates the rules used to decide whether an action performed on the Concept Keyboard is a click, double-click or pressed action. The time delay values should be:
   $t < 0.15$ sec $t' < 0.6$ sec $t'' > 1.1$ sec.
When a pressed action has been detected, a beep sound is emitted.

Direct manipulation

All commands are accessible by means of keys on the overlay. Simple rules were adopted to allow an intuitive understanding of the commands and to facilitate their memorisation.

For instance, the location of a read command corresponds to the objects to be read. As shown on figure 5, all buttons on the left part of the overlay are *read-the -line-in-front-of-me* commands, whereas buttons on the top are *read-the-column-above-me* commands. Clicking, double clicking or pressing the read command buttons address the different sounds that objects can emit.

The cut, move and copy commands are activated by
   1- pointing and clicking on an object,
   2- pointing and clicking in the right location - if necessary - and,
   3- pointing and clicking on the command button.

The system responds by enunciating the action to be performed. The user can then confirm the command by double-clicking the command button.

Since all interactions rely on concrete and sensitive objects, simplified sets of user commands and rapid feedback, this interface corresponds to the general definition of direct manipulation (Verplank, 1988). This definition can thus be extended to non-visual direct manipulation.

Sounds

Both sampled sounds and synthesised spoken messages were used. Their duration had to be chosen carefully depending on the type of activity to allow clear identification or comprehension but also to avoid being a load. We also adopted the principle that if an action was to involve a sound utterance, any sound in progress was to be stopped.

Semantic organisation

A systematic semantic organisation of messages was adopted which means that the message associated with the click action can usually be described as giving a concrete and immediate aspect of evoked reality. The double-click sound generally provides more sophisticated information. The pressed sound can be a meta-message. An example should make this clear. Let us imagine that the object to be evoked is a cat. The messages associated with its location could be:
   click action: "miow" resulting from a sampling operation,
   double-click action: "My name is Pussy"
   press action: "A cat is a domestic animal, it lives in a house with people".

Use in the classroom

As long as a device has not been used extensively in real conditions, no conclusion can be drawn about its adequacy to the objectives for which it was designed. An experiment was therefore carried out for about a year with both visually impaired and sighted children in two schools in the Parisian suburbs. It involved about 20 students ranging in age from 6 to 10 years, i.e. CP, CM2 in the French system. Among the visually impaired several were totally blind. Students worked in small groups of 3 or 4. Training sessions took place once a week and lasted about 40 minutes. This section gives some examples of activities that were organised using Tactison.

Little Noise's Family

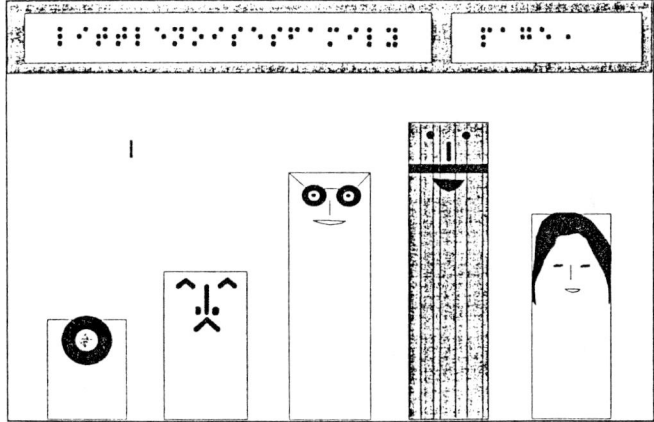

Fig. 7. Little Noise's Family Overlay. Characters are stylised. Simple tactual conventions simplify their identification. Neither mobile objects nor commands are provided.

Little Noise is a character used to introduce the TactiSon system. He and his family were central to many activities presented to the children. These characters turned out to be very useful in creating a motivating environment. Little Noise has a sister, called Melody, a brother called Wordy, father and mother. Melody has a canary bird which appears as a very short raised line on the overlay.

The training sessions using this overlay were also aimed at introducing prerequisite basic concepts and functioning rules. Particular emphasis was placed on spatial verbalisation. Depending on their age, children were taught or rehearsed the opposition between left and right, close and far in order to locate the corresponding parts on the horizontal surface of the overlay. They were also trained in how to click, double-click and press.

Scrambled animals

After checking that basic concepts and manipulations have been mastered, more complex activities can be proposed. Figure 8 shows an example where students are asked to classify objets by moving them from one box to another. The reasoning is as follows: Little Noise loves collecting animal pictures. Naughty Wordy dropped two image boxes into the bin. Little-Noise has to put them back into their original boxes. To solve this problem, children have to learn operating commands and explore a set of disordered objects. It is worth noting that the visual perception of this overlay appears quite orderly, quite different from the corresponding haptic and auditory perceptions. This is because not all locations in the bin contain objects and because lines and columns of patterns are not as noticeable when explored by touch.

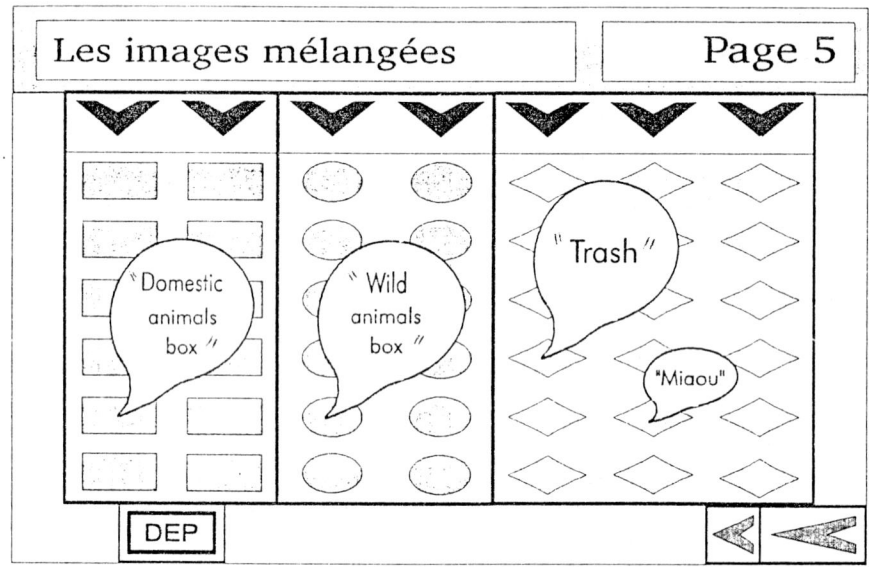

Fig. 8. Scrambled Animals Overlay. It illustrates how messages can give indications to the users

Sentence Construction

Figure 9 shows an overlay designed for an exercise based on the manipulation of lexical material. A box contains words which have to be used to build sentences. It functions in a similar way to the previous overlay. This underlines how the same basic functioning principles can find quite different teaching applications.

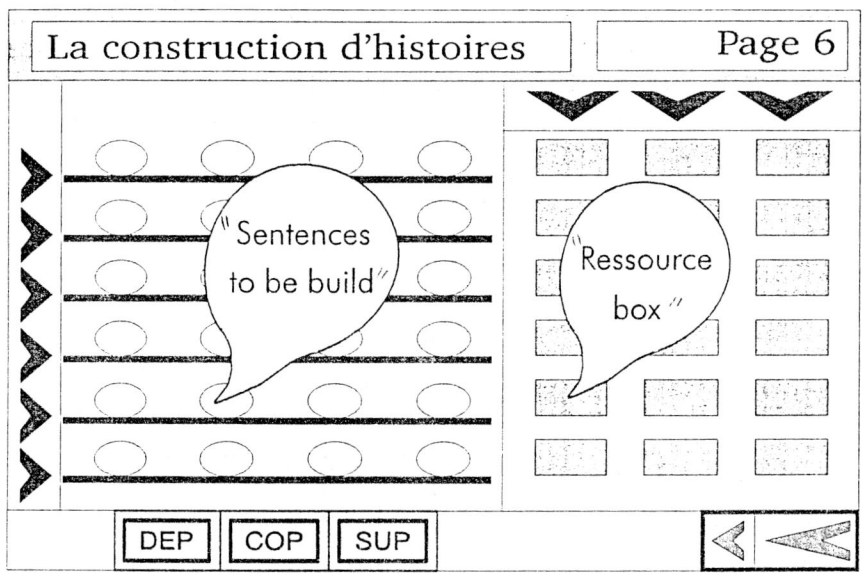

Fig. 9. Sentence Construction Overlay.

DISCUSSION

Because of the many aspects that are involved, the thorough evaluation of any learning tool is a difficult and probably never-ended enterprise. Pedagogical, psychological, and ergonomical aspects have to be taken into consideration. Moreover, keeping one aspect apart from the others, or isolating a parameter often makes no sense at all. Does this mean that it is not possible to evaluate learning tools?

In fact, one has to distinguish two levels in the evaluation of learning tools. First, low-level, rather general questions can be addressed in a first evaluation step. Questions are of the following type: *Does it work properly? Does it stimulate active attitudes among children? Does it offer a wide variety of possible applications?* But also: *What skill or ability does it address? In what sense is it new? What kind of exercise does it allow that was not possible before?*

Our experiment suggests that only a few, well devised and carefully prepared training sessions can answer such questions satisfactorily. Both teachers and students appear to be quite reliable experts.

In a second step, evaluation has more precise aims which are more difficult to accomplish. The questions concern the causal relationships between an exercise implemented on the learning tool to be evaluated and the acquisition of a given notion or about the efficiency of this exercise compared with a more traditional one.

The following section is intended to provide some insights on first evaluation step of TactiSon resulting from the experiment carried out for a total of 20 hours training in several groups.

Three points of view will be given: that of students, that of teachers and that of the designers. They cover three general concerns. How appealing is the system? How does it fit in with pedagogical objectives? How could it be improved?

The students' point of view

- The first point to come out of the experiment was the eagerness with which children participated in the weekly Tactison training sessions. This type of medium was quite new to them. The discovery of the auditory contents of the overlay was a source of fun and often entailed frolics. It sometimes appeared like a game of hide-and-seek. Charlotte, age 7, would exclaim "My goodness, there is somebody in here". Peter, age 9, said "Let's have fun and put the phone in the bin".

- Children learned to operate the device very rapidly. All were perfectly able to master the three different actions, i.e. click, double-click and press, within the first hour of training. Aurélie, age 6, even suggested "One could also have a triple-click!". They immediately understood the semantic organisation of the messages attached to the different types of actions.

- The situations created with TactiSon entailed brisk debates among students. For example, the scrambled animals activity entailed an argument about the definition of domestic as opposed to wild. On that occasion, it was decided that an elephant can be either wild (in the African jungle) or domestic (helping people in India).

- Another important point to be reported is that the metaphor of mobile objects underneath the overlay was accepted without any difficulty. For instance, Jane, age 8, said "Let me see something in here. I wonder whether the panther is still here" Then Aurélie: "There is no one here any more because the animal has gone". Jane: "Never mind, I will find it and put it back".

- Most of the time students were able to work quite autonomously. Navigation commands on the right of the overlays allowed them to pass from one exercise to another which meant obtaining the appropriate overlay. Nevertheless, this sometimes lead to mismatch errors.

The teachers' point of view

- Teachers appreciated the facilities dealing with different presentations of the same concept. The example has already been given of the different types of messages that can evoke a cat. Other aspects can be emphasised depending on the pedagogical aim: spelling, locating a word depending on the class to which it belongs, its texture depending on its functional value.

Thus, auditory and haptic transitory sensations are used to contribute to the construction of more global and permanent representations of a concept. This is of great importance for the education of the blind, particularly since the overuse of verbal exchanges without connection to sensorial experiences can lead to inadequate attitudes when facing real situations, known as verbalism.

- They also pointed out that this type of device offers rich opportunities to make children aware of spatial organisation and to train their ability to think about space. This point is of prime importance since it often appears to be a bottleneck in the education of the blind.

- The possibility that was given to students to move and organise objects within boxes was also prized as "an excellent way of training logic skills". It was considered as "more practicable than manipulatives since it does not weigh 2 kg and since objects cannot be lost or thrown down".

- Many applications were suggested, including exercises and games which involve various types of material, such as letters, words, numbers, notes and melodies. For instance, a crossword puzzle was especially designed for TactiSon.

- Activities were principally organised in groups. All the participants were provided with their own overlay, but only one leader student was in charge of interacting with the device. However, in order to make the situation useful for participants who could not see the manipulation in progress, the leader had to explain precisely to others what he or she was doing. Such communication rules had to be imposed, or preferably, adopted after discussion. They took advantage of the weakness of feedback on this point to enrich the pedagogical situation in order to make it useful in other similar situations that are very common among groups of visually impaired .
- Last but not least, they expressed a strong need for authoring tools which help them to create new exercises.

The designers point of view

This point of view can be divided into observations and prospects:

Observations

- The design rules emerging during this study were very specific and rarely obvious. Once a solution had been tested out, it became a kind of standard for future interface design. Such rules also concerned tactile diagrams, sounds and interaction methods.

Three concrete examples can be given:
a) the localisation and identification of Melody's canary bird was generally very quick, often quicker than for other characters. This appears contrary to what visual experience suggests.
b) regular layout in rows and columns does not evoke such an orderly organisation when explored by hand compared with vision.
c) as explained above, feedback messages are emitted before actions have been performed while in visual interaction feedback is obtained by observing the moving image on the screen. This exemplifies how non-visual interaction sometimes has to be designed in a very special style.

• Despite the fact that speech production was obtained through a high-quality speech synthesiser, the variety of voice timbres appeared very poor, presenting some difficulties for some exercises. On the contrary, pre-sampled sounds were greatly appreciated by children.

• The number of different messages attached to an object has often been questioned. Despite the absence of proof, the number three seems to be a rather convenient figure, related to what children were able to manage simultaneously.

Prospects

• The addition of a braille output would be easy and would enrich opportunities to train reading and spelling skills.

• Automatic identification of the overlays, possibly by means of bar-coded marks or other techniques, could improve the interface by making the choice of page more natural.

• Commands allowing the transformation of sounds or even recording and editing facilities should be added in order to make the system more flexible. Nevertheless one has to keep in mind that any enrichment of the set of commands will increase their number and thus make the interface more complicated. Gestual dialogue mixed with speech recognition techniques could be useful in tackling this problem (Burger, 1992).

• Techniques presented at this conference could soon reinforce the metaphor and probably make it closer to reality. For instance, recent research makes it possible to think of enhanced input devices that would give the user a dynamic feedback about the location of objects. Thanks to gesture recognition, input actions such as pinching and seizing gestures could be used to move sounds as if they were concrete things.

• It is worth noting that the presentation adopted for mobile objects may find a more professional application by making the desktop metaphor more accessible to the blind.

• An authoring tool should cover the following need : the creation of tactile overlays, sound recording and editing, and the design of exercises, i.e. audio-tactiles and functions. Obviously its interface should offer either visual or non-visual dialogue facilities !

CONCLUSION

The projects that we have been carrying out over the last few years, in particular TactiSon, have led to encouraging conclusions concerning the development of technological learning environments based on non-visual modalities, i.e. audition, touch and proprioception. These environments should be rich enough for teachers to consider them useful complements to existing techniques. It is hoped that multimodal non-visual interfaces will help close the gap between the richness of learning materials available for the sighted and the relative scarcity of those accessible to the blind. There is no doubt that it constitutes a challenge, but it is also a motivating reason for elaborating co-operative research projects associating special-need teachers, psychologists, neuroscientists and engineers.

REFERENCES

Burger D. and Suchard J. (1991), SoundBench : a HyperCard Program for Blind Children. *Interactive Multimedia*, 2(4), p.5-15.

Burger D., Beltrando E. and Sagot J. Sound Synthesis and Bar- code Technology to Develop Learning Environments for Blind Children. *Journal of Visual Impairment and Blindness*, 84, p.565-569.

Burger D., Liard C. and Roux G. A sound-based learning tool for both blind and sighted children. In : *proceedings of the IEEE/ Engineering in medicine and biology society Ninth Annuel Conference*, Boston, 13-16 novembre 1987, p.2026-2027.

Burger D. La multimodalité : un moyen d'améliorer l'accessibilité des systèmes informatiques pour les personnes handicapées. In : *Actes de ERGO-IA 92*, Biarritz 7-9 octobre 1992.

Fraiberg S. (1977), *Insights from the blind*, New York : Basic Books.

Schneekloth L.H. (1989), Play Environment for Visually Impaired Children. *Journal of Visual Impairement and Blindness*, 83, p.196-201.

Hinton R. (1991), First introduction to tactiles. *The British Journal of Visual Impairment*, 9(3), p.79-82.

Parkes D. (1991), Nomad: enabling access to graphics and text based information for blind, visually impaired and other disability groups, in *Proceedings of Worl Congress on Technology for People with Disabilities*, Washington DC, December 1-5 1991, p.689-716.

Keiras D.E. & Bovair S. (1984), The role of mental model in learning to operate a device, *Cognitive Science*, 8, p.255-273.

Verplank W.L. (1988), Graphic challenges in designing object-oriented user interfaces, in *Handbook of Human-Computer Interaction*, M. Helander (ed.), Elsevier Science Publishers, North-Holland, p.365-376.

Résumé

Les sons constituent un élément important du monde qui nous entoure. Ils nous aident à interpréter bon nombre d'événements survenant autour de nous. Dès l'enfance, la modalité auditive joue un rôle essentiel dans l'apprentissage.

L'objectif de cet article est d'examiner l'apport possible des technologies nouvelles pour la réalisation de matériels pédagogiques interactifs fondés sur l'audition et accessibles à de jeunes enfants, en particulier aveugles ou déficients visuels. Tout d'abord nous rappelons l'efficacité du support papier. Nous passons ensuite brièvement en revue les matériels pédagogiques traditionnellement utilisés avec des enfants déficients visuels. Enfin nous présentons différents systèmes développés par les auteurs et expérimentés dans différentes écoles, grâce auxquels les élèves peuvent manipuler des sons comme les pièces d'un jeu de construction sur une table de jeu. Ces exemples nous semblent illustrer comment les technologies nouvelles permettent la création d'outils pédagogiques ne reposant pas sur la modalité visuelle et pourtant aussi faciles à utiliser et aussi riches que peuvent l'être les images traditionnelles.

Construction of New Interfaces

There seemed to be no use in waiting by the little door, so she went back to the table, half hoping she might find another key on it, or at any rate a book of rules for shutting people up like telescopes: this time she found a little bottle on it, and tied round the neck of the bottle was a paper label with the works «DRINK ME" beautifully printed on it in large letters.

Lewis Carroll

"Natural Input/Output is the ultimate user friendly interface. It places the burden of the communication squarely on the computer rather than on human".

Maureen Caudill
(Byte april, 1992)

Prospects for objects and standards in the interaction between computers and blind users

Jean-Claude Sperandio

Université René-Descartes, Paris V, 28, rue Serpente, 75006 Paris, France

ABSTRACT

Improvements in the ergonomics of graphic interfaces and their widespread use over the last few years is undeniably a good thing for users. However, graphic interfaces are not standardised and contain many non-textual components, mixed with textual elements. Therefore, developers of blind-oriented interfaces have difficulties in extracting from graphic interfaces all elements (in ASCII code) that can be pronounced or spelt by a vocal synthesiser or displayed on a braille terminal.

Advances in graphic interface standardisation could improve homogeneity between applications and new software architectures, thus facilitating the design of new interface layers which could be adapted for blind users. Standardisation of multimedia systems could also benefit the development of blind-oriented systems.

A short summary of the standardisation of graphic interfaces and multimedia devices is given. Advantages and disadvantages of braille terminals and of voice synthesisers are presented. We underline the lack of theoretical and practical knowledge about presenting visual forms and objects which are usually displayed on screens in a non-visual way. We also stress the lack of basic and pluridisciplinary research on non-visual perception and on the mental representation of physical objects by blind users.

INTRODUCTION

One of the most obvious advances in current computer technology involves the increasing importance of computer-user interfaces, in particular graphic interfaces (called GUI, Graphical User Interface). In these interfaces, figures, graphics, diagrams, icons, buttons, etc., are displaced on a colour screen, together with texts or numbers in movable, elastic and superposable windows.

In general, graphic interfaces are "object-oriented": the user can directly manipulate objects (files, devices, controls, etc.) by using a mouse or other such device to point to the image of these objects displayed on the screen. This direct manipulation sets off a series of commands with rapid feedback, rather than the traditional line of commands in an unnatural language.

According to Verplanck (1988), "direct manipulation user interfaces are now becoming widespread because of the availability, at a reasonable cost, of three key enabling technologies: 1) raster graphics, especially bit-map displays, for the presentation of complex images, 2) pointing devices, especially the mouse, for rapid analogic input, and 3) computing power dedicated to reacting dynamically and meaningfully to the user's actions".

Standards and special tools designed to develop such interfaces are increasingly widespread. The hope is to facilitate their development, to improve both software portability to different machines and homogeneity between existing interfaces which may be used by the same user, and also to improve the ergonomic quality of man-computer dialogue, tailored to the requirements of particular tasks and users.

Graphic interfaces with direct manipulation have the reputation of being easy to learn and use, of being interactive and of containing the functions that allow people to do the things they want to do and that are well liked. However, whereas this technological progress may be undeniably a good thing for most users, it is not the case for the blind. It has made the situation even worse. The current solution for blind users consists in "capturing the screen", i.e. in picking up all ASCII characters that it is possible to read and then in recoding them, either tactily on a refreshable braille display or auditorily with voice synthesis. These options are appropriate with classical alpha-numeric interfaces, but not with WIMP interfaces (Windows, Icons, Menus, Pointer) in which many elements are non textual, and thus not directly readable.

Consequently, the problem has to be approached in a different manner. Instead of trying to read the screen, it is necessary to delve into a deeper level of the software, below the screen interface, and to build over this deep level (i.e. the computational kernel) with a new interface, especially designed for blind users. Don't forget that information is fundamentally symbolic, first coded with numerals for computer processing purpose, and then coded in a certain way depending on the displays.

Developers of devices especially adapted for the blind hope that the standardisation of some aspects of software applications or devices will reduce the number of technical difficulties encountered during their development. Surely. However, both the current lack of standardisation in software and hardware products, and problems with software architecture create difficulties for the design of non-visual interfaces for blind users. New methods of programming recommend a strict separation between the kernel and interface. This separation is essential with multimedia interfaces. Therefore, the development of special interfaces for blind users is directly concerned with multimedia standards.

We will now present the state of the art of visual interfaces and multimedia devices, continually underlining the fact that standardisation is still limited and heterogeneous.

STANDARDS FOR VISUAL INTERFACES

Smith, a pioneer in user-interface standardisation, recalled (in op. cit., 1988) that "in the past, tools were tailored to their users, ...[but] with the industrial revolution and the development of mass production, we have come to rely on more uniform design and more formal design standards". Standards can follow two general purposes: a technical quality improvement (i.e. the optimal choice, according to experts) or a consensus between competitors (i.e. one choice accepted by most competitors in order to provide a certain compatibility of hardware and software).

Terminology (norms, standards, recommendations, guidelines, requirements, specifications, etc.) is inconsistent between authors and countries. Smith (1988) has distinguished four terms:
- "design standard, a series of generally stated requirements for user interface design, imposed in some formal way, e.g. by legislation, by contract, by management decree, etc."
- "design guidelines, a series of generally stated recommendations for user interface software, with examples, added explanation, and other commentary, selected (and perhaps modified) for any particular system application, and adopted by agreement among people concerned with interface design".
- "design rules, a series of design specifications for a particular system application, stated specifically so that they do not require any further interpretation by user interface software designers".
- "design algorithms, computer programs implementing (and imposing) design rules, which may control automatic generation of user interface software".

And Smith wrote (in 1988!) that "such algorithms are only now beginning to be devised, but they will become more common in the future". This prediction is now coming true.

In France, several ergonomic norms have been created by AFNOR, the French organisation for standards. The goal of ergonomic norms is to protect users or workers from the poor design of products, tools, work stations, buildings, etc., in relation to criteria such as safety, health, fatigue, comfort, etc. A major interest of norms for user-computer interfaces is to help developers improve design, for example to avoid a badly fitting interface with, for instance, too few characters, a bad choice of colours, too long menus, unmeaningful icons, bad structure of texts or data, etc.

Another advantage of norms is to provide a greater degree of homogeneity between applications, in order to facilitate the learning of new interfaces. Generally, users do not read technical booklets of each application and expect that a new interface behaves like other interfaces. Since user's habits are a "second nature", similarity and homogeneity of interfaces should be respected by developers whenever possible and convenient. The well-known Macintosh interface system is a good example of homogeneity and consistency.

An example of an ergonomic norm related to software design is the recommendation AFNOR n Z 67.110 (January 1988) entitled Ergonomie et conception du dialogue Homme-Ordinateur (Ergonomics and design of Man-Computer Dialogue). In most countries (USA, GB, Germany, France, etc.), official ergonomic standards are provided on hardware or software aspects. At an international level (ISO), a standard entitled "Ergonomic requirements for office work with visual display terminals (VDTs), n ISO 9241", is expected very shortly. This standard deals with software aspects of man-computer dialogues and describes precisely many practical items which apply seven main general principles:

- suitability for the task,
- self-descriptiveness,
- controllability,
- conformity with user expectations,
- error tolerance,
- suitability for individualisation,
- suitability for learning.

This ISO standard is not only limited to graphic interfaces, but deals with all software aspects of work on visual display terminals. Nevertheless, this standard does not deal with non-visual interfaces and we are not aware of an equivalent ergonomic standard for non-visual interfaces, in particular for blind users. The document specifies (part 10) that "this international standard provides ergonomic principles which are formulated in general terms, i.e. they are presented without reference to situations of use, applications, environments, and technology. These principles can be used in the design of dialogue systems and in their evaluation".

It is obvious that this kind of standard is a set of recommendations, it may be useful, but it is not law. The text is pedagogic, but software designers and developers will probably consider it too general. However, these ergonomic principles are now more and more accepted in developers' culture. Therefore, we can see these principles implemented (more or less) in the design of new interfaces. A story initiated with the coming of Macintosh ...

Another, more efficient kind of standard is not set by experts, but imposed by the market. These standards are not official, but result from the product or the scale of products strongly integrated into the market and are generally sponsored by a leader or by a union of influent companies. This is typical for standards dealing with graphic interfaces and multimedia devices.

Standards of WIMP interfaces determine both the interface look that the user sees on the screen, and the basis objects (called widgets) displayed on the interface and handled by the interface manager. Widgets and basic procedures used to handle them are defined and handled according to particular principles and tools. Basic tools (in toolkits) and the interface manager above them are specific to each Operating System.

Thus, due to the fact that a given toolkit is designed for a given Operating System and that WIMP interfaces require a fast processor and a large amount of central memory, standards of graphic interfaces are not just a set of principles available for all machines, but they are closely connected with the hardware.

Standards of WIMP interfaces are divided into three technological "computer worlds" (Fig. 1):

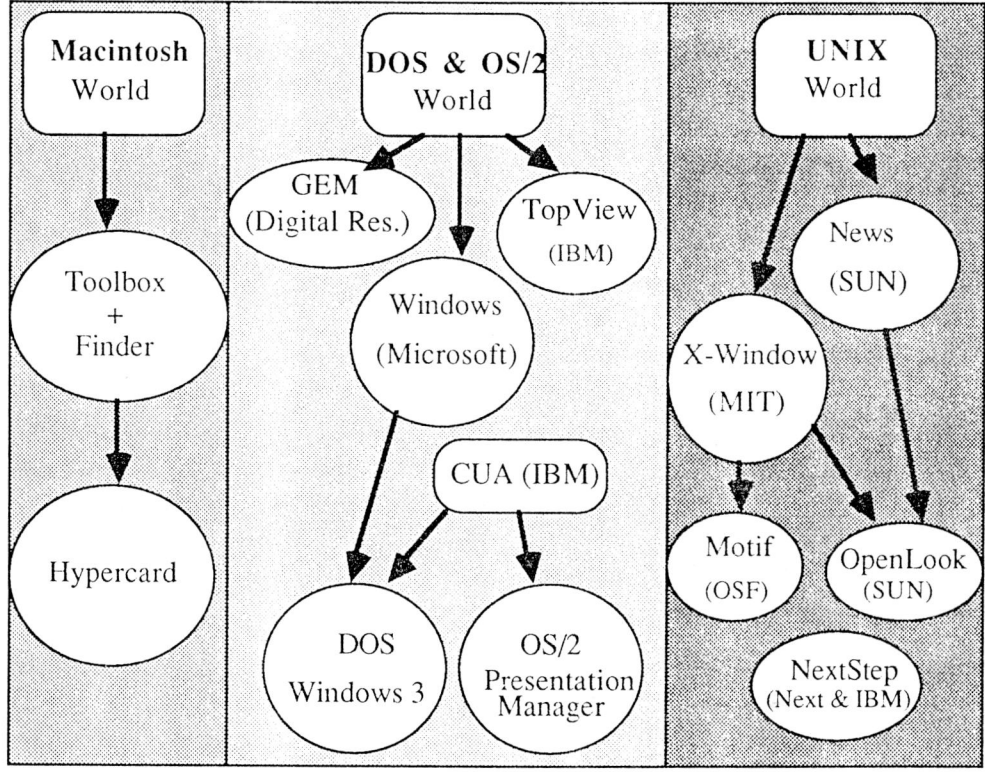

Fig. 1: *Graphic Interfaces Standards (adapted from Meinadier, 1991.*

The Apple World

This interface is entirely designed on a single standard, the Macintosh, on sale since 1984, heir to the Lisa in 1983, itself heir to the Star of Xerox in 1981. Clearly defined in an object-oriented programming philosophy, the interface is supported by the MacOs (Operating System of the Macintosh), the Finder (the manager of files and windows) and the Toolbox which has greatly expanded over the years. From the outset, this standard benefited from the high performances and qualities of the Motorola 68X00 microprocessor, and by a precise graphic screen.

The Toolbox of the Operating System is accessible by all programmers, a fact which results in a high level of homogeneity between all designed interfaces. From an ergonomic point of view, the usability of this interface is a reference for competitors.

The IBM-PC World (and other compatible computers)

The Operating System MS-DOS, designed by Microsoft for the Intel 8088 microprocessor, is infamous for it poor usability. Nevertheless, this family of microcomputers has been sold widely. Since 1984-85, three graphic toolkits and window manager systems have been developed: namely TopView by IBM, GEM by Digital Research, MS-Windows by Microsoft.

These three systems were inspired by the Macintosh look and feel, but have not been as commercially successful. However, TopView has been the base-plate of the future standard CUA (Common User Access) developed by IBM in 1987. The first implementation of the standard CUA was Presentation Manager in 1988, a system which is both a toolkit for programming interfaces and a windows manager for enhanced IBM PCs on OS/2. The major advantage of CUA is to provide general guidelines for writing graphic interfaces, based on ergonomic principles and implemented in a concrete system. In 1990, Microsoft adopted the standard CUA for the new version of Windows 3.1 on DOS for microprocessors Intel 80286; 80386 or 80486.

To sum up, we can say that the connection between IBM and Microsoft makes CUA a standard de facto (though CUA is not enhanced or innovating with regard to the Macintosh look and feel, from which its main features are borrowed). CUA is thus doubly implemented, by Microsoft with Windows 3.1 and by IBM with Presentation Manager on OS/2.

The UNIX world

Unix, of which there are several versions, in particular Unix System V from AT&T, and Unix SBD from Berkeley University, is the Operating System of most "work stations". The first implementation of a graphic interface system on Unix was NeWs (Network Extensible Wondowing System) designed and developed by SUN, a leader in the work station market.

More recently, Next Computer developed NextStep, a graphic interface which, like NeWs, uses Postscript, the graphic language developed by Adobe for printing, and Display Postscript for screen displays.

But the origin of a real standard for graphic interfaces on Unix is X-Windows. Designed in 1985 by MIT in the Athena project, commercialisation dates from 1988. Several versions followed including the famous Version 5 in 1991. Open Desktop is an X-Window version developed by SCO. X-Windows contains a basic library (X-Lib) in which there are dialogue functions, and a normed protocol of exchanges according to a customer-server mode (X11 Wire Protocol).

However, X-Windows is not a toolkit, it is a model and a frame of interface architecture and does not impose a particular look and feel, but leaves developers free to build their own toolkit and window / file managers. Therefore, many toolkits have been built on X-Windows and the X11 protocol, but two toolkits are now prevalent and compete with one another for the status of standard de facto: Motif and Open Look.

Motif was developed at the end of 1989, sponsored by OSF (Open Standard Foundation) which groups IBM, DEC, HP, Bull, Microsoft, etc. Motif thus combines various elements from the members of this union, in particular Motif adopts the IBM/CUA look and feel. Therefore a Motif interface is quite similar, in look and feel, to a Windows 3.1 interface or a Presentation Manager interface.

Open Look was also developed in 1989 by SUN and Unix International partners (the union rival of OSF). Open Look is built in part on NeWs, but uses the X-Windows protocol (X11). The look and feel of Open Look is thus also similar to Motif.

Thus, the current trend seems to be towards the unification of products or more exactly the combination of parts of several leader products. For example, the next enhanced version of Windows NT from Microsoft will keep the look of Windows 3.1, but will take into account the functionalities of Motif on Unix and will be implemented indifferently on various microprocessors. MOOLIT (MOtif and Open Look Intrinsic Toolkit) will be a toolkit which would allow developers to design a Motif and an Open Look version of the same application simultaneously.

Beyond these standards, which obviously promote a certain homogeneity of products and applications, development tools, in particular interface builders, play an increasingly prominent unifying role. These tools can be divided into three categories: toolkits, application skeletons and interface builders.

A toolkit is essentially a library of basic objects (widgets) with functions and procedures to handle these widgets, at a low level. Several examples have been mentioned above.

An application skeleton is a frame built over a toolkit from which basic resources are borrowed. It is a frame, a canvas of interfaces which are parametered, expandable and reusable, from which the developers derive concrete interfaces, modifying or expanding some aspects while deleting others. Several examples are mentioned in [Coutaz 90]: Apex, Grow, Serpent, MacApp, etc.

An interface builder is a program creating concrete interfaces solely from a set of specifications. The developer, or also a non programmer, draws the interface features, places widgets and windows on the screen and links them to functions and procedures. Various kinds of interface builders have been developed, with many differences, in particular:
- the language used to specify the interface,
- the language used for commands and its own interface (ergonomic),
- the language used to program functions and procedures for handling widgets,

- the operating system and the kind of connected hardware,
- the more or less extended toolkit,
- the imposed or non imposed standard, only one or several.

Examples of interface builders are: *Aïda /Masaï* from Ilog (France), *Interface Builder* from Next Computer, *HP-Architect* from HP, *Xface Maker 2* from NSL. Etc.

STANDARDS FOR MULTIMEDIA DEVICES

As mentioned above, current standards for computer-user interfaces deal with visual interfaces and especially with graphic interfaces. For several years, computers have been used for handling not only numbers, texts or widgets displayed on screens, but also sounds, schemas, drawings, photographs, video images, etc. Entries are not only from keyboards or mice, but from many very different devices. All these objects form the multimedia world which requires a certain standardisation in order to provide a minimum level of compatibility between devices.

Specialists in ergonomics consider that multimedia man-computer communication is a substantial improvement over the screen-keyboard monopoly. It can not only enlarge the set of objects to be manipulated, processed and displayed by computers, by also to enlarge the repertory of man-computer dialogues. Limits and disadvantages of screen-keyboard dialogues are largely known and expounded in ergonomics, not just for visually impaired users.

In the multimedia world, - which is a wide commercial battle-field -, all current standards are issued from commercial unions or more or less imposed by the leadership of an influent manufacturer or software developer.

Standards deal with particular kinds of devices (CD-ROM, CD-TV, CD-I, CD-Photo, Video Cards, Audio cards, etc.), and also with the software linked to these devices. Currently, several manufacturers' unions exist, with IMA (Interactive Multimedia Association) dominating since 1988. IMA unites about two hundred members (Sony, Philips, Kodak, IBM, Apple, Microsoft, ...). There are also other more or less rival unions or coalitions who aim to share the market and provide standards. For example: MPC (Multimedia PC), TWAIN (a set of requirements for integrating images on PC and Mac), Kaleida (a joint-venture IBM/Apple), - (Taligent is another joint-venture IBM/Apple) -, JPEG (Joint Photographic Experts Group), MPEG (Motion Picture Experts Group), H261, etc.

The development of multimedia interfaces also requires special toolkits and tools. Some of these tools are extended from graphical interface tools, a few are really innovating, for example using hypermedia concepts and technics, such as Hypercard (from Apple), one of the first and simplest multimedia system builders.

PERSPECTIVES FOR BLIND USERS

Why are blinds users interested in standards for visual interfaces or for multimedia systems? Firstly, because some multimedia devices are directly usable by blind users, such as sounds, audio documents, CD-ROM, etc., but the main reason is that with multimedia technologies, each medium is a particular world and a standardisation of deep levels of software is required in order to provide possible communication between these different worlds. This is particularly important for developing products devoted to blind users. Classical interfaces, particularly graphic interfaces, are screen-oriented and thus current applications are also screen-oriented. Multimedia applications are (or will be) programmed with intent to support, simultaneously or not, various media. And why not include media adapted to blind users?

New concepts are interesting on this score. The concept of an object itself can first be seen as a concrete entity (for example, a widget displayed on the screen, as a text, an icon, a menu, etc..., or a word displayed on a braille window, or a sound, etc., but an object can also be seen as an abstract entity which does not imply a particular aspect, but can be represented in various forms on various media. Object-oriented programming is more than a method or a philosophy. There are object-oriented languages, O-O interfaces, O-O Operating Systems, etc. For example, the DOI (Document-Oriented Interface) is a recent new interface concept built around the concept of object. According to Cary Lu (1992), "DOI computing is the logical culmination of the object-oriented revolution. It provides a natural way of interacting with the daunting world of objects. ../.. The DOI is an advanced user interface that makes documents, not applications, the focus of personal computing".

The DOI is task-oriented and allows access to applications through documents. In a DOI interface, each object communicates with other objects by sending and receiving information by messages in a form that other objects and tools can understand. The aspect of an object is a particular property (or a property of the class) and can be modified, as well as the support (medium), without modifying messages addressed to it. An interesting idea in the DOI is that the interface is chosen according to the task and can be changed according to users. This is possible only if the interface implementation is absolutely separated from the computational kernel of the application.

The "separation principle" between the deep levels of the application and the superficial levels of the interface requires an adequate architecture. It is necessary, not only for blind-oriented interfaces, but also for any multimedia interface. A multimedia interface implies multimodality and provides users with a greater choice of input / output channels. For the blind, it provides the possibility of communicating with computers by means of auditory, tactile and/or audio-tactile modes.

DIFFICULTIES OCCURRING IN VISUAL-TO-NON-VISUAL TRANSLATION. INTERDISCIPLINARY CONJUGATION

If we suppose that all technical problems can be solved (for example, by a good architecture of applications, by new interface concepts, or by consistent advances in standardisation!), the idea, interesting for devices especially devoted to blind users, is to generate a specific interface directly over the kernel of the application, instead of "capturing" the screen.

But another, perhaps greater difficulty remains: Which medium should be used? What non-visual forms of these objects can be designed to replace the visual forms? How can audition and tact be mixed and used in parallel? What is the role of haptics in interactions with computers?

Answers to these questions require a scientific and pragmatic knowledge of non-visual perception and of non-visual data processing by humans, particularly by the blind. Despite a lot of very beautiful studies in cognitive psychology on the blind, particularly on the blind infant (see Hatwell in this volume), my opinion is that there is still a lack of fundamental knowledge about many aspects of non-visual perception and other cognitive functions linked with perception. On blind adults, some recent studies (several of which are presented by speakers in this conference) have been carried out on the use of voice synthesis, braille refreshable displays and other tactile devices, but that is not enough. In psychology and in ergonomics, many studies have been carried out on visuo-tactile coordinations, but only a few on audio-tactile ones.

It is obvious that current blind-oriented devices such as braille terminals and voice synthesis are very useful but are limited.

A braille terminal is a kind of window with a span of 20, 40 or 80 characters, each allowing tactile perception by a finger and thus a possible decoding if the user knows braille. Not all blind people know braille! Such a device is relatively expensive (for only a small screen), only allows slow reading and users must move the span frequently. Moreover, the braille code has 6 points giving 64 possibilities, instead of the 256 possibilities of ASCII. There are extended braille codes with 8 points, but they are not normalised. Perhaps normalisation could begin by the extended braille code itself! Texts displayed on screens are enhanced by various attributes such as colour, italics, bold-faced types, underlining, etc., these attributes are generally lost in braille recoding.

Voice synthesis, like braille windows, are also limited to texts. There are now various systems in different languages which, at a reasonable cost, provide a relatively good vocal quality, including functions such as continue reading, word to word reading, spelling, stop and return, etc. Some defects remain, for example: imperfect prosody, defective pronunciation of some words, monotonous speech, mediocre ergonomics of controls, etc. Nevertheless, voice synthesis is currently the device most able to compete with the screen. Differences concern reading speed, but more fundamentally reading strategies. Audition, and thus voice synthesis, is necessarily linear, contrary to vision which allows browsing anywhere in the visual field.

Tactile perception also allows a certain amount of browsing, but tactile devices at the present time have too limited a surface, at least at a reasonable cost. The span of braille terminals is low compared with the screen. In fact, voice synthesis and tactile devices (braille windows) are complementary and can be included on the same device with a consistent control system.

We are now in the field of texts, which are consequently readable. But, how can we recode non-textual objects which are currently coded visually on the screen? How can non-visual coding be used, for example, for a curve, a graph, a schema, a photo? Is it possible to code these things other than visually? Could these kinds of objects be perceived by a sensory modality other than vision? If it is possible, what computer technology or electronic solutions should be used or designed? An interesting job would be to list the series of requirements of a satisfactory coding which could replace visual coding on screens.

Pointing to objects on a braille terminal is not impossible, although very difficult. And with voice synthesis? Direct manipulation of objects, like in graphic interfaces, normally requires a spatial display, a suitable pointing device and visual feedback. Some visual objects, for example icons or items in menus, can be checked auditorily, but not without difficulty. Time is to audition what space is to vision. Icons are generally labelled with a name and thus it is easy to translate a set of icons into a list of names that can be read by voice synthesis. However, there are many differences between visual reading and listening. Visual readers can read and process the list as they like. The spatial structure of the list, which may be a multi-level tree, and possible enhancements are salient. On the contrary, the listener depends on linear listening. If an adapted control is provided, the listener can stop the enumerated list at any point, but first this action is not very precise and second structure and enhancements are lost or impoverished. The challenge is to provide a system which preserves all information.

Another well-known object of visual interfaces is the window. Windows provide to the visual user with an immediate structure for objects and data displayed on the screen. A window can contain other windows or structured objects, such as dialogue boxes or templates. It is possible, sometimes not without technical difficulties, to pronounce or spell texts displayed in windows, but how can the two-dimensional structure borne by windows themselves be translated?

Several speakers during this conference will answer some of these questions by presenting some technological advances as well as some scientific knowledge concerning, for example, cognitive aspects. For example, mathematical formulas, graphs and curves can be displayed by means of sounds (see Edwards & Stevens in this volume). Icons can be displayed by means of earcons. In some measure, images and drawings can be displayed on tactile and/or audio-tactile devices (see Hinton in this volume). And so on. This means that research is in progress, but we have to underline that contributions from several competences are required.

First, blind users have an irreplaceable experience. Research teams associate this experience with their own scientific or technical competence.

Evidently, competences of computer specialists or electronics specialists are required, not only to develop technical solutions, but also to invent and test new devices. We also need competences of psychologists, experts in perception, particularly in non-visual perception. Psychologists and psychophysiologists have carried out less research on non-visual perception than on visual perception. Even auditory perception has been studied less than visual perception, studies are less numerous, less thorough and often more specialised on a particular field, such as for example music. This lack of knowledge is also underlined in ergonomics.

We need inventiveness and we have to explore new ways. For example, research carried out in Montreal by Martial and Dufresne (1992) on sound-icons has provided musical forms instead to visual icons, to be associated with different semantics.

Psychologists have meticulously studied the visual reading of texts. Reading tables, schemas, pictures, etc. has been studied, but much less than texts. Auditory reading, for example by means of voice synthesis, has been studied very little. Visual or non-visual reading includes various strategies answering questions such as: "Is this text (or this object) interesting for me?" (and not only: "what is written?"). "What are objects (figures, photos,...) inside, imprecated with the text?" "How is the text displayed: in lines, in columns in paragraphs, etc.?" Although these attributes are visual, a non-visual access may eventually be possible.

Even less is known about tactile perception than auditory perception. Interesting investigations have been carried out on braille reading (with one hand, with two hands, on a book or on a 20-, 40-, 80-window, etc.), but other research is required, particularly when braille reading is associated with voice synthesis. Braille reading is not the only way of using human capabilities of tactile perception.

Mental representations are also involved in perception. For example, the place of metaphors in the computer world is well known, particularly in interfaces such as the "desktop metaphor". Martial and Dufresne (1992) investigated whether or not this desktop metaphor is available for blind users, as it is for other users. The ergonomic method used by these psychologists was to observe blind people at home or in their office. Do blind and other users arrange their desks in the same way? What kind of "mental picture" of their office do blind person have? (workspace, objects, tasks as goals and subgoals, actions linked to tasks). What kind of perceptual conditions allow the blind to build a mental model and operate on it? Are differences relevant with regard to the desktop metaphor (like that used in graphic interfaces)? Martial and Dufresne's results have confirmed a previous study of Lie (1985): although the spatial organisation of office desks of late blind subjects is very similar to that of congenitally blind subjects and differs from that of normally sighted people, the mental representation of late blind subjects is more similar to that of normally sighted subjects than of that of congenitally blind subjects. In particular, Martial and Dufresne wrote that late blind subjects, like normally sighted people, attempt to visualise mentally the environment and their memory seems to be visual rather than tactile or auditory. I think that this conclusion will not surprise Y. Hatwell!

Last year, Karine Gornet, a member of our research team, carried out an experiment on listening to texts displayed by a voice synthesis (i.e. auditory reading). Three groups were compared: late blind, congenitally blind and normally sighted subjects. Texts varied in length and complexity. Subjects had to explore these texts and to understand them. Free browsing was allowed and browsing strategies were observed and analysed. Subjects then had to answer questions about texts. Results did not show significant differences between groups, but did show some suggestive differences between subjects, independent of blindness.

Among inter-disciplinary competences, I have not forgotten ergonomics. Ergonomists provide methods for analysing tasks and users, and for evaluating new devices, with an experimental approach, either in the laboratory, or preferably directly in the field (cf. above, Martial and Dufresne). Ergonomists like to choose experimental tasks, scenarios and performance criteria in order to apply scientific results, rather than to investigate fundamental aspects of cognitive behaviour. Ergonomists are firstly interested in evaluating new devices in real life conditions or, better, in designing new systems. A good design of blind-oriented systems requires a precise analysis of specific needs of the blind in the office or at home and an investigation of specific difficulties in using computers and other tools.

CONCLUSION

Some years ago, human-computer dialogues were very poor, and then visual interfaces were developed which were mainly limited to texts. Graphic interfaces have become increasingly complex. Multimedia devices are just being born. Therefore, a technical and conceptual gap between visual and non-visual communication with computers is not surprising.

For the blind, multimedia technologies are an opportunity and a hope. The program of this symposium and the panel of invited speakers have, for ambition, to draw up the current state of the art of various aspects among different technical and scientific specialities, but also to suggest new tracks for research.

REFERENCES

Coutaz J. (1990), *Interfaces homme-ordinateur. Conception et réalisation*, Dunod Informatique, Paris, 455 p.

Gornet K. (1992), Les stratégies de lecture auditive chez les voyants, les aveugles tardifs et les aveugles de naissance au cours d'une tâche de recherche d'informations, *Mémoire de DEA Psychologie des Processus Cognitifs*, Université Paris V, septembre 92.

Lie I. (1985), On replacement and problem solving potentials of spatial aids for the blind, In *Electronic Spatial Sensing for the blind, contributions from Perception, Rehabilitation and Computer Vision*, D.H. Warren & E.R. Strelow, Riverside, California, p.391-401.

Lu. C. (1992), Objects for end users, *Byte*, december 1992, p.143-152.

Martial O. & Dufresne A. (1992), Pour l'accès aux interfaces graphiques par les non-voyants: analyse des représentations mentales du bureau, *Actes du coll. ERGO-IA '92*, octobre 92, Biarritz, France, p.278-290.

Meinadier J.P. (1991), *L'interface utilisateur. Pour une interface plus conviviale*, Coll Informatique et stratégie, Dunod, Paris., 222 p.

Smith S. L. (1988), Standards versus guidelines for designing user interface softwar, in *Handbook of Human-Computer Interaction*, M. Helander (ed.), Elsevier Science Publishers, North-Holland, p.877-889.

Verplank W.L. (1988), Graphic challenges in designing object-oriented user interfaces, In *Handbook of Human-Computer Interaction*, M. Helander (ed.), Elsevier Science Publishers, North-Holland, p.365-376.

Résumé

L'amélioration de la qualité ergonomique des interfaces graphiques au cours des dernières années, ainsi que leur large diffusion, constitue un incontestable progrès pour les utilisateurs. Ces interfaces, cependant, souffrent d'un manque de standardisation et comportent de nombreux éléments non textuels mélangés aux éléments textuels. De ce fait, les développeurs d'interfaces pour aveugles ont quelque difficulté à extraire les composants (constitués de caractères ASCII) pouvant être prononcés ou épelés par une synthèse vocale ou recodés sur un afficheur braille.

En revanche, les tendances de standardisation auxquelles on assiste actuellement devraient améliorer l'homogénéité de la programmation et conduire à choisir des architectures d'applications sur lesquelles pourront être plus facilement greffées des couches d'interfaces adaptées aux aveugles. La standardisation des systèmes multi-média devrait également être bénéfique pour le développement de systèmes pour aveugles.

Après une courte synthèse de la standardisation encore partielle des interfaces graphiques et du monde multi-média, une réflexion est amorcée sur les avantages et inconvénients des afficheurs braille et des synthétiseurs, en soulignant le manque de savoir-faire théorique et pratique pour présenter non visuellement des formes et des objets que nous sommes habitués en informatique à présenter sur des écrans. Le besoin en recherches fondamentales et pluridisciplinaires sur la perception d'objets non visuels et sur la représentation du monde physique par les aveugles est exprimé.

Software solutions to the problem of GUI inacessibility to blind persons

Jane Berliss

Berkeley Systems, Inc., 2095 Rose Street, Berkeley, CA 94709, USA

ABSTRACT

Computer interface design has undergone a massive revolution in the last ten years. The Graphical User Interface (GUI), which has influenced popular platforms such as Macintosh and Microsoft Windows, goes beyond text to convey and organize information through pictorial metaphors, e.g., icons, trash cans and folders. While this interface is proving more accessible to blind people than was originally thought, there are still problems in making sure blind people have full access to the power of GUI-based computers. This paper outlines the history, state of the art, and probable future of ensuring this full access, with a particular focus on ways that different developers can share the same base technologies.

"When one thinks about advances in computer architecture and accessibility by persons with disabilities, it is useful to remember that the Chinese symbol for crisis is the symbol for danger combined with the symbol for opportunity." Boyd et al. (1990)

INTRODUCTION

In early 1984, Apple Computer introduced the Macintosh, the first mass-market computer based on a *Graphical User Interface (GUI)* operating system. The average consumer had little difficulty noticing the distinction between the Mac interface and the interface of more traditional systems. Perhaps the most notable feature was that the screen was deliberately designed to draw on metaphoric references to familiar objects: trash cans for throwing away files, folders for organizing files, and so forth. These metaphors were primarily accomplished via *icons* - small pictures that represent the intended image. Glancing at these icons alone would convince most sighted users that here indeed was a revolution in human-computer interface. In addition, the use of a hand-held device, called a *mouse,* for the first time permitted the cursor to be moved randomly to any part of the screen and on-screen objects to be physically re-arranged.

Because developers used a heavily visual design metaphor, it was assumed that blind people would never be able to access GUI systems. Yet not only can these systems be made usable, there are even many features of the GUI that have particular advantages for blind users. For example, GUIs are developed with a set of rules that, when followed by third-party developers, provide for wide consistency among applications, reducing the need for memorizing commands. In addition, almost all applications have pull-down "menus" listing commands; these menus are available to the user at all times. Finally, applications and system-level information appear in adjustable-size boxes called "windows." It is possible to have multiple windows open simultaneously, making it easy for users to move between applications and still be able to quickly access system-level functions.

However, the GUI does pose specific access problems for blind people. Designers of GUI systems have assumed that all users would have a high level of hand-eye coordination for mouse use, the ability to see and recognize icons, and the ability to move the cursor automatically to any given area of the screen. Although the screen—reading program *outSPOKEN* and the Optacon interface program *inTOUCH* have provided workable Macintosh access solutions based on, respectively, speech and tactile outputs, the blind user still cannot take complete advantage of GUI systems. Since these systems are becoming increasingly predominant in the educational and work environments, blind people will need to have full access to them to remain competitive. Even though other systems continue to exist, blind computer users should always have the choice to use GUI systems for whatever reasons are important to them.

There have been a variety of access models proposed for making sure that blind people have access to the power of GUI-based systems. Some have been built on existing models for access to text-based systems; e.g., use of specifically-designed applications (word processors, databases, etc.) that can share files with mainstream applications (Burger, 1992). Others have tried to consider the GUI as a unique access problem/opportunity, and to develop access models accordingly. This paper explores the history of the latter approach, and surveys both current implementations and proposed solutions under investigation.

ACCESS TECHNIQUES

Figure 1 demonstrates the two major differences, and accompanying access problems, between text-based systems and the GUI. The first difference, pixel-based screen rendering instead of direct-to-screen text mapping, has been dealt with via development of an off-screen model (OSM). The second difference, which is a set of human-computer interaction strategies that rely heavily on visual metaphors and abilities, is far more complex (Boyd *et al.*, 1990).

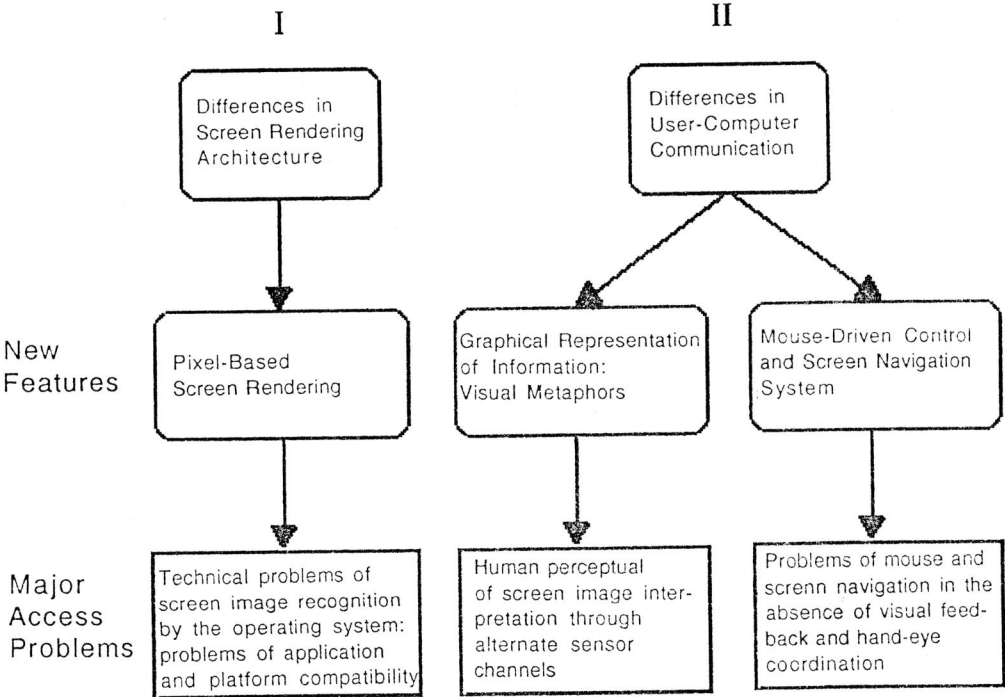

Fig. 1: Major differences between the graphical user interface and traditional user interfaces, with general categories of features and access problems for blind users. Adapted from: Boyd, L.H. et al. (1990).

The OSM works as a database for capturing information that is both visible and not visible on-screen. It retains a high level representation of text, icons, symbols, controls, and other information that would otherwise merely be a collection of pixels. In addition, the OSM captures essential information such as cursor location and font size and style. OutSPOKEN, a Macintosh screen reading program released by Berkeley Systems in 1989, contained the first commercially-implemented OSM, and projects such as IBM's Screen Reader for OS/2 and the Trace Center's Systems 3 research prototype have also used OSMs.

The graphic-based interface was designed under the assumption that users would be able to see and interpret on-screen information and would have sufficient hand-eye coordination to use the mouse. This alone has proved problematic for some sighted users - e.g., users with some types of learning disabilities, or even those who for whatever reason do not understand metaphors such as deleting a file by moving it to a picture of a garbage can. Blind users have the additional difficulty of being able to use neither the screen nor the mouse; they must retrieve and enter information through some other means. These means have to date centered around mouse emulation and simple speech and tactile output, which have not always provided full access. For GUI-based systems to become truly accessible to blind people, therefore, it has been necessary to look at solutions that take all elements of a graphical user interface into account - dialog boxes, icons, etc. - and present them in a way that blind people find not only useable but also truly meaningful.

NEW ARCHITECTURES

In the mainstream, a major model for the development of graphic-based operating systems has been the *Seeheim model*, created at a German workshop in 1982 (Bass et al., 1991). Figure 2 shows the Seeheim model for development of *user interface management systems (UIMSs)*. According to this model, the user interacts directly with a Presentation Component, while the data structures and routines required by the computer are in the Application Interface Model. The "dialogue" between user and computer is managed by the Dialogue Control (Green, 1985).

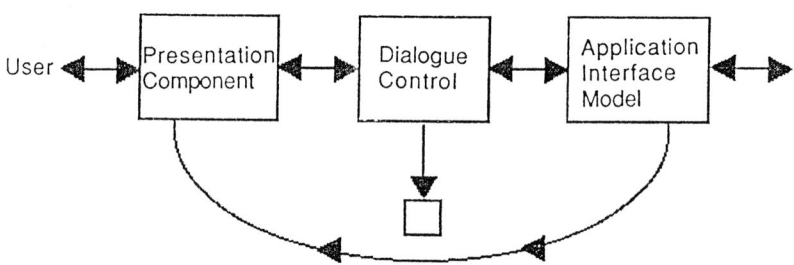

Fig. 2: The components of a user interface. Adapted from: Green. M. (1985), The University of Alberta user interface management system, Computer Graphics, 19(3), p.206. Cited in: Bass, Len et all. (1991).

In time, the Seeheim model was found to be inadequate, in that it failed to sufficiently describe the necessary complexity of both the Presentation Component and the Application Interface Model. In response, the *Arch model* (Fig. 3) was developed. This model adds an Interaction Toolkit Component to the Presentation Component to describe the portion of the GUI that interacts directly with the operator. It also divides the Application Interface Model into a Domain-Specific Component (which implements user-independent functions) and a Domain-Adaptor Component (which mediates between the Dialogue and Domain-Specific components).

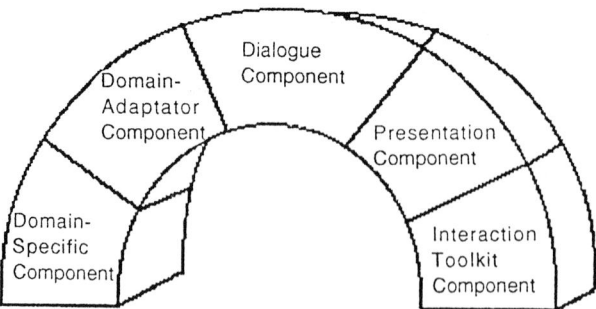

Fig. 3: The five components of the Arch Model. Adapted from: Bass, Len et al. (1991).

Various objects and structures are developed from these components; these serve as interfaces for transmitting information between components (Fig. 4). Because some systems involve more than one implementation of one or more components, the model has been further expanded to illustrate branching (Fig. 5) (Bass *et. al.*, 1991).

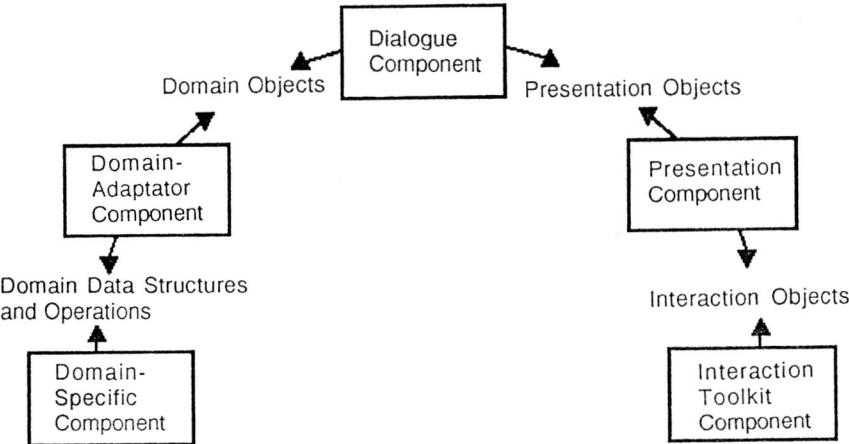

Fig. 4: The interfaces between the components. Adapted from: Bass, Len, et al. (1991).

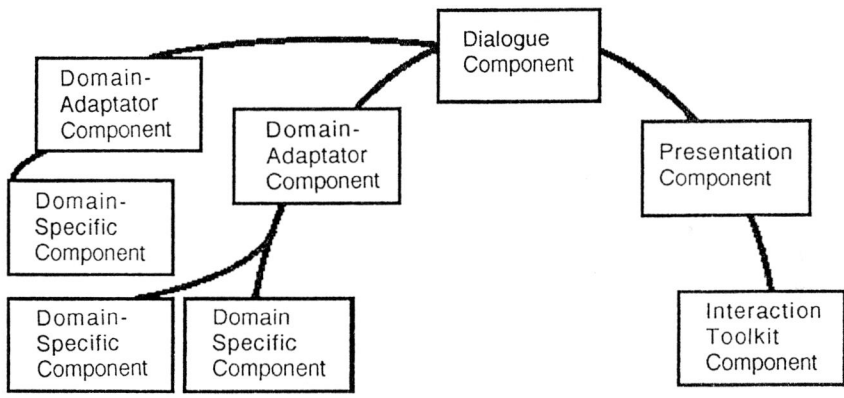

Fig. 5: Example of branching with multiple Domain-Specific Components. Adapted from: Bass, Len et al. (1991)

Stephanidis *et al.* (1991) discuss design criteria for non-visual user interfaces. They propose two strategies for providing access: a toolkit for translating visual primitives into meaningful non-visual primitives, and a UIMS that would allow users to choose between "sighted" access and "blind" access at the system level. The bulk of their paper is devoted to exploring this latter strategy.

Unfortunately, while the idea of a "multiple access" UIMS makes good sense, it is unlikely to be implemented. A tremendous amount of effort would be needed to convince mainstream computer manufacturers to put development effort into accommodations for what is likely to be perceived as an insignificantly small number of users, despite the argument that sighted users would benefit from use of auditory and tactile access (Stephanidis et al., 1991). Even if this were accomplished, it would take additional time and effort to ensure that the UIMS was constructed correctly. Blind people need access to the systems that exist today to remain competitive in the employment and academic arenas, and need quick access to new systems as they are released. At this time it appears most practical, if not necessarily optimal, to develop separate, third-party solutions for meeting the needs of blind users.

COLLECTION OF DATA FROM THE GUI

Currently, access to GUI systems by blind users is accomplished by taking advantage of one or both of two senses: hearing and touch (the latter via tactile representations of graphics and text and/or Braille translation of text). The former has been predominant, since speech-output strategies require less expensive hardware and a much shorter learning curve than tactile strategies.

Boyd et al. (1990) created a model of four levels of access to GUI systems, to be achieved in three stages (Figs. 6, 7). The levels move from specific to universal compatibility with operating systems and applications, from difficult to simple modifiability, and most importantly from low to high levels of access to GUI functionality by blind users. These levels are realized by moving from software-based solutions with limited GUI compatibility to solutions that use a wide range of equipment.

Within this model, there is tremendous potential for creativity. One recently marketed solution is *An Open Book* from Arkenstone, Inc. An Open Book builds on Arkenstone's existing Optical Character Recognition (OCR) strategies to create a unit that is essentially a computer and an OCR device with a full-page hand scanner in a single unit. As Arkenstone president James Fruchterman points out, "Not only do [hand-scanner based] systems hold the promise of cost decreases, but they also offer a far better portable solution than hitherto has been available" (Fruchterman, 1992).

Another innovation in access to the GUI is *Systems 3*, a tactile device currently in prototype stage being developed by the Trace Center in Madison, Wisconsin. Systems 3 consists of a standard graphics tablet, a T-shaped mouse-puck with a tactile array and mouse-emulating buttons, and driver software.

When Systems 3 is connected to a computer, the user can move the mouse-puck across the tablet and feel the information (graphics, icons, etc.) in the corresponding virtual location on the screen. A speech output component activates whenever text is encountered and reads this information aloud. This project is designed to enhance access to graphical information (Vanderheiden and Kunz, 1990).

Level 1 Access
General
Restricted to one operating system and one application.
Difficult or impossible for third parties or individuals to adapt to new situations and needs.
Specific
Can recognize and manipulate standard text in highly specialized and isolated situations.
Level 2 Access
General
Restricted to one operating system, applies to a wide range of applications.
Specific
Can recognize and manipulate standard text.
Can recognize icons and simple graphics.
Can recognize pull-down menus, windows, pop-up dialogue boxes, buttons.
Can move around the screen and manipulate screen objects (without the mouse).
Limited ability to scan and browse screen information.
Limited ability to perceive locational and contextual (formatting) screen information.
Level 3 Access
General
Easily adapted across operating systems.
Applies to most applications and easily adaptable to special cases.
Specific
Can interpret some standard computer graphics (e.g., bar graphs, pie charts).
Can use the mouse and pointer for orientation, navigation, and control.
Can scan and browse screen information.
Can perceive locational and contextual (formatting) screen information.
Level 4 Access
General
Applies across all operating systems and all applications.
Allows third-party developers and individuals to modify to fit special needs and new situations.
Specific
Provides all the functionalities of the graphical user interface at the same levels as for sighted people.

Fig. 6: Levels of access to the graphical user interface. Adapted from Boyd, L.H., et al. (1990).

Stage 1

Seeks Level 1 Access
Restricted to one operating system.
Usually a customized approach for one application.
Limited to interpreting standard text.

Based primarily on software.
Based primarily on one adaptive aid: screen reader or Braille translator.
Based primarily on one alternative sensory channel: speech output or Braille.

Stage 2

Seeks Level 2 Access
Restricted to one operating system.
Applies to a wide range of applications.
Interprets standard text, simple icons.
Can recognize and manipulate windows, etc.
Navigates by keystroke navigation system.
Limited browsing and format perception.

Based primarily on software.
Based primarily on one adaptive aid: screen reader or Braille translator.
Based primarily on one alternative sensory channel: speech output or Braille.

Stage 3

Seeks Level 3 and Level 4 Access
Maximum operating system independence.
Compatibility with all applications.
Can interpret graphs, charts, and complex drawings.
Full browsing and locational capabilities.
Full mouse control.
Supplementary voice input control.
Easily modified by third parties and individuals.

Uses both software and hardware.
Modifies and integrates adaptive aids.
Integrates multiple nonvisual communication channels: speech output, voice recognition, tactile, haptics, and auditory cues.

Fig. 7: Major features of access Stages 1, 2, and 3. Adapted from Boyd L.H., et al. (1990):

It would be extremely difficult - and, most likely, undesirable - for any single developer to create access solutions to meet all user needs and preferences. Since access solutions at Levels 3 and 4 of the Boyd model are designed to be maximally applicable across operating systems, it follows that there is a need for the multiplicity of developers to work cooperatively and efficiently to implement these solutions. In particular, there is no sense in having to continually reinvent OSMs and other cross-platform code if a standard set of code can be made available via a developers' toolkit.

ACCESS TO PRESENT AND FUTURE OPERATING SYSTEMS

GUI Access, the developers' toolkit created by Berkeley Systems of Berkeley, California, is one implementation of a third-party toolkit strategy. This toolkit permits development of access solutions at Level 3 of the Boyd model, and facilitates dissemination of technologies such as the OSM.

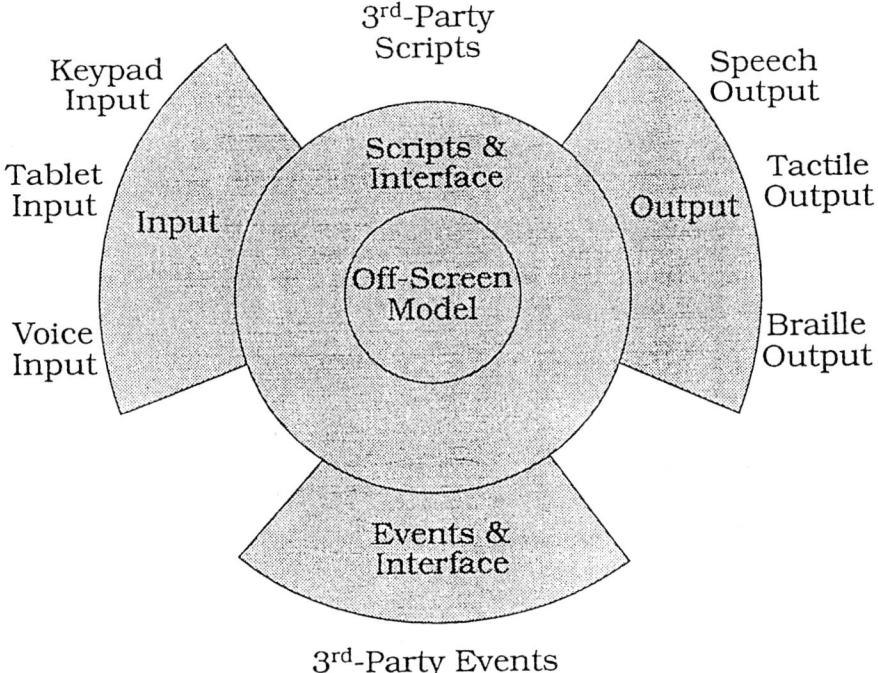

Fig. 8: GUI Access—functional diagram. From: Korn, Peter & Drees, Ben (1992).

Figure 8 shows a functional diagram of GUI Access. To explain its workings in terms of the Arch model, GUI Access captures information in the Off-Screen Model (OSM) at the Domain-Specific level. *Scripts*, which are executable routines that tend to be linked into the toolkit at the Interaction Toolkit level during runtime, can be used to carry out functions such as extending the basic navigation capabilities of GUI Access and further configuring alternative input or output devices. *Events*, which tend to be Presentation Components such as dialog boxes, may also trigger execution of a script, such as moving the mouse to the upper left corner of the box. Input and output drivers (Interaction Objects) are added to the basic toolkit to permit use of alternative devices for entering and retrieving information (Korn and Drees, 1992; Bass *et al.*, 1991).

As with the Arch model, GUI Access is structured to permit multiple implementations of one or more component categories. Figure 9 shows a sample of how GUI Access might be applied. Input from one or more standard or alternative (e.g., speech input) devices is sent to the core GUI Access technology, where it may interact with scripts and/or events. The resulting information is sent to one or more standard or alternative (e.g., Braille display) output devices. This structure facilitates development of Stage 3 Access according to the Boyd model (Korn and Drees, 1992).

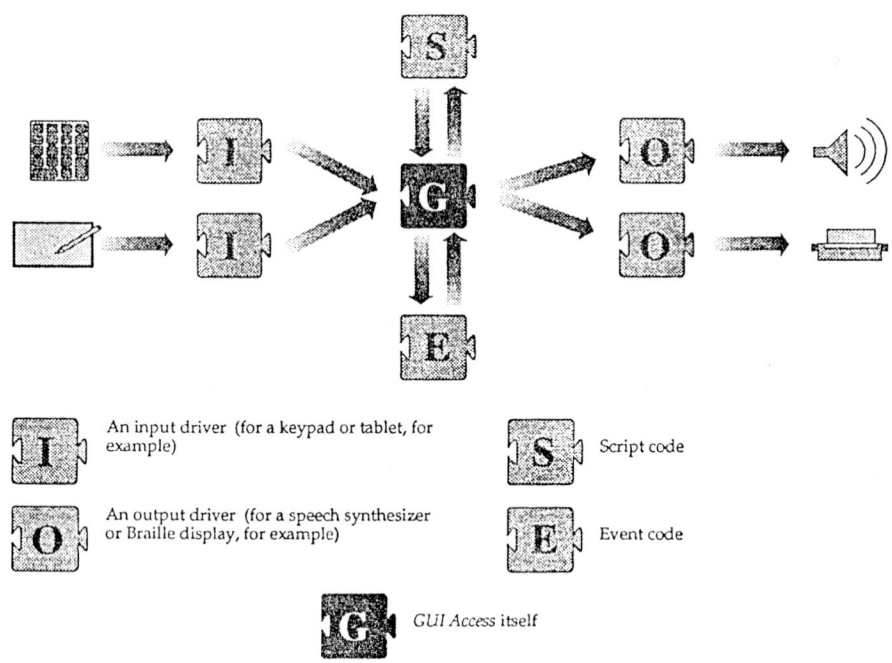

Fig. 9: GUI Access - a sample application. From: Korn, Peter, and Drees, Ben (1992).

GUI Access is deliberately designed so that as much code as possible is platform-independent. The base technology can be used not only for multiple access strategies, but also for solutions that can be adapted, with minimal programming, across multiple platforms. This means that, as new GUI platforms are released, access strategies can be quickly developed and made available; in turn, blind individuals will be able to learn and use new platforms almost as quickly as their peers. Figure 10 shows which portions of the toolkit are platform independent and which are platform dependent, and indicates what code needs to be developed by third parties.

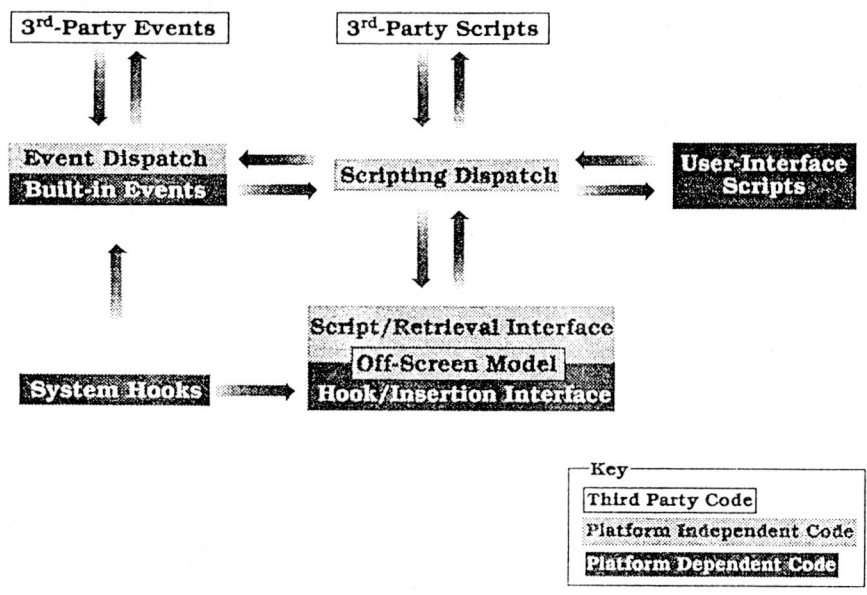

Fig. 10: GUI Access core modules. From: Korn, Peter, and Drees, Ben (1992).

GUI Access is seen as a dynamic product, especially since it does not yet permit Level 4 access according to the Boyd model. For example, not all mainstream programs follow the rules for compatibility with a specific GUI. This is especially true for programs originally developed for text-based systems and then ported to a GUI version. It also affects "flexible" authoring tools, such as HyperCard for the Macintosh, which allow developers or even end-users to create applications that use an infinite number of variations on the system's GUI. Because existing access solutions assume compliance with GUI development standards, any deviation from these standards will cause access problems that may or may not be insurmountable with GUI Access. The only foreseeable solutions are to convince application developers that they need to follow GUI development guidelines whenever possible, and to continue using toolkits such as GUI Access to explore access solutions.

ACCESS SOLUTIONS IN EXPLORATORY/PROTOTYPE STAGES

An exciting facet of access research is finding new strategies for conveying information through the senses of hearing and touch. One particularly intriguing concept is that of *three-dimensional sound*, i.e., sound that conveys not only what the on-screen information is, but also where on the screen it is located. In January 1993, Advanced Gravis announced the release of *UltraSound 3D*, which "processes the audio signal through a technique called convolution, where new right and left binaural audio signals are generated that create a wraparound sound effect to the human ear. The sound signal is a stereo signal shaped electronically to make the listener hear the sound as three-dimensional and in the correct location — a psychoacoustic effect that can be manipulated in real time..." (Advanced Gravis, 1993). In other words, blind users could receive auditory cues that the cursor is at the top of the screen, is being moved from right to left, etc. This technology holds great promise for providing further assistance in screen navigation.

Other innovative approaches are currently being explored for future implementation. One of the most creative is *stereotypic image interpretation*. This involves taking predictable images, such as certain types of charts or graphs, and automatically creating a small table that describes the image. The user can then query the table to elicit specific information about the image (Vanderheiden, 1991).

Even with these ideas, however, there remain some problems for which a satisfactory solution has not yet been adequately proposed. One issue that needs further research is that of multiple disability. For example, the primary cause of non-congenital blindness in the United States is diabetes, which also causes a reduction in tactile sensitivity. There is not yet a system for providing computer access should a blind diabetic also have or acquire severe hearing loss - a distinct possibility within a rapidly aging society. While fingerspelling mechanical hands hold some limited promise, more work needs to be done to determine the best solution to this access issue.

CONCLUSION

While the GUI Access toolkit has been created in consultation with several computer manufacturers, no single tool can ever be the last word in providing access. GUI-based systems will always be predominantly aimed towards the majority, sighted population, and any number of factors may make current access strategies quickly outdated. What is more important than any individual approach is continued dialogue among mainstream manufacturers, access specialists, and above all blind users and potential users of GUI-based systems, many of whom are still unaware of even the current level of GUI accessibility.

REFERENCES

Advanced Gravis (1993), *Advanced Gravis — Software 2: Product Seen*, Press Release.

Bass Len & al. (1991), *The Arch Model: Seeheim Revisited*, User Interface Developers' Workshop

Boyd L.H. & al. (1990), The Graphical User Interface: Crisis, Danger and Opportunity, *Journal of Visual Impairment and Blindness, 84 (10)*, p.496-502.

Fruchterman J. R. (1992), Reading Machines, *Paper submitted for the Technology & Reading/Learning Difficulties conference*, San Francisco, January 16-18 1992, 11 p.

Korn P. & Drees B. (1992), GUI Access: a Developers Toolkit, *Application Programming Interface (API) report*. Berkeley Systems, Inc., December 1992.

Schwerdtfeger R. S. (1991), *Making the GUI Talk*, Byte, December 1991, p.118-124, 126-128.

Stephanidis C. et al. (1991), Access to Graphical User Interfaces by blind people, *Concerted Action on Technology and Blindness*, May 1991, p.1-65.

Vanderheiden G. C. & Kunz D. C. (1990), Systems 3: An Interface to Graphic Computers for Blind Users, *Proceedings of the RESNA 13th Annual Conference*, Washington, D.C., p.259-260.

Vanderheiden G. C. (1991), *Graphic User Interfaces: A Tough Problem with a Net Gain for Users Who Are Blind*, Technology and Disability, 1 (1), p.93-99.

The author wishes to thank Bo Gehring, Gregg Vanderheiden, Peter Borden, James Fruchterman, Dominique Burger, Marc Sutton, Josh Miele, and especially Tracy Edgecomb, Peter Korn, and Ben Drees for their assistance with this paper.

Résumé

Les systèmes d'interface ont connu au cours des dix dernières années une révolution importante avec l'arrivée massive des interfaces en mode graphique ou GUI (Graphical User Interface). Les logiciels de large diffusion conçus pour des environnements tels que le Macintosh d'Apple ou Windows de Microsoft utilisent largement des métaphores visuelles dans lesquelles on identifie, par exemple, des icônes, des dossiers, une corbeille à papier.

Rendre de telles interfaces accessibles pour les personnes aveugles apparaît finalement moins difficile qu'il n'avait semblé au départ. Cependant, certains problèmes restent à résoudre pour que ces personnes puissent bénéficier pleinement de la puissance des applications reposant sur les interfaces graphiques.

Cet article rappelle l'historique, l'état de l'art et envisage le futur prévisible des développements destinés à améliorer l'accessibilité des applications informatiques pour les personnes aveugles. Il examine et discute en particulier les méthodes de conception des logiciels susceptibles de fournir une base technologique commune à différents développeurs de solutions adaptées.

Trends in human-machine multi-modal interaction

J.C. Martin[1][2] and D. Béroule[1]

[1] LIMSI, BP 133, 91403 Orsay Cedex, France, [2] ENST, 46, rue Barrault, 75634 Paris Cedex 13, France

ABSTRACT

Human-machine interaction may involve several input and output communication channels which are combined so as to exhibit coherent behaviour. Interaction is then called "Multimodal". Although it results in more natural interactions and other advantages, multimodality is shown to add its own set of problems to those already posed by monomodal systems, such as the real-time co-ordination of modalities, their fusion, segregation and skill acquisition. Illustrative multimodal systems which deal with these questions are presented. Finally, a real-time computational architecture based on coincidence detection is proposed as a possible approach to multimodal dialogues.

INTRODUCTION

There he is, in front of M^3, the Multi-Modal Machine which is supposed to help him design interactively the plan of his future house. Nobody has told our architect apprentice how to use this fantastic tool. No User's Guide is available; "not necessary" they said. Amazingly, the relationship he just entered into with the machine gives no indication of misunderstandings, even fewer than in some human-human dialogues...If the machine utters a technical term, and notices the user hesitate, the written form of the word is displayed, together with a drawing of the corresponding object enhanced in the current plan. Conversely, the machine is able to learn new words, taking advantage of both current context and spelling information provided by the user through the keyboard. In the top right-hand corner of the screen, a little funny face expresses the message currently being synthesised, in order to facilitate its comprehension through lip reading. Written messages are displayed close by. But most of the screen is devoted to the plan plotting task, performed by the user via a choice of tools such as a mouse or a touch screen. An impressive feeling of three-dimensional space is created by a couple of loudspeakers, with variable balance, intensity and reverberation. While a piece of furniture is shifted from one room to another following a spoken request, with a mouse click showing the destination ("move the table here"), a characteristic creaking sound may be heard.

The loudspeaker balance corresponds to the location of the movement for a virtual listener situated at the bottom of the screen, whereas reverberation provides information concerning the room's volume and the distance separating the listener from the moving object. Some people say that even the visually impaired can use M^3, provided that specific acoustic feedback is generated by the machine while users try to follow the screen plan contour with fingers in order to refresh their "mental image" of the current house plan. The feature of M^3 preferred by users is the ability to keep its artificial ears continually open, especially while synthesising speech. Volume increases when the environment gets noisy. It may decide that its explanation is not clear and shift to another, possibly bringing into play another modality. Although computer interfaces involved in this friendly interaction are already available, M^3 still belongs to science-fiction. But how far are current systems from this ideal machine? This matter will first be considered through the presentation of general problems raised by human-machine interactions and specific problems related to multi-modality. Solutions to these problems are then illustrated by current realisations. A different research framework is then presented, based on coincidence detection and aimed at resulting in a homogeneous computational architecture.

MULTI-MODAL HUMAN-MACHINE COMMUNICATION

Main problems in human-machine interactions

With the advent of the use of natural communication, such as speech or gestures, a new problem arises which did not exist when computer interfaces were limited to discrete inputs, such as those delivered by a keyboard. The change from continuous to discrete signals constitutes a crucial point to be addressed by the system, which determines its global efficiency. For instance, continuous speech must at least be segmented into words, which involves syntactic information together with the detection of physical features of the signal. It may even be segmented into syllables, phones or discrete spectral events (Calliope, 1989). This requirement also applies to the automatic recognition of gestures (Bradffort et al., 1992; Teil & Da Silva, 1991).

While interacting with a machine, we send signals with significant time courses (acoustic speech signals, keyboard inputs, signals corresponding to a movement detected via a dataglove). A human-machine communication system should take into account this temporal aspect, especially if it is aimed at treating several modalities at the same time. Asynchronous messages should be treated in real-time in order to preserve the natural quality of dialogues.

Another problem with natural signals comes from their complex, variable and unpredictable nature, which does not leave the machine designer the possibility of modelling them fully *a priori*. These signals must be acquired during the life-time of the machine, so as to store labelled reference patterns in its memory. For the purpose of recognition, these references may then be compared with unknown input patterns. The reference closest to the input provides a label. Although often separated from the actual "recognition phase", the acquisition of internal references, referred to as the "learning phase" should really work continuously whenever unexpected events occur in the machine environment, without being under user supervision.

Further, pattern inherent variability requires that different occurrences of the same pattern should be taken into account for shaping "prototypical" internal representations of this pattern. This is a main argument in favour of continuous learning. Anyhow, variability may express itself in so many ways that a significant part of the recognition procedure is devoted to this question. Temporal variation, associated, for instance, in speech with several possible pronunciation rates, is dealt with rather accurately by digital Dynamic Time Warping algorithms (Calliope, 1989).

A last and main problem to be addressed when dealing with natural continuous signals remains unsolved, apart from in a few restricted cases. Extra uninteresting signals are often present in the device input stream, from which a single significant signal must be extracted and identified. In speech processing, stable background noise can be subtracted from the total input. But noise is especially disturbing and hard to work with when made of speech items or unexpected accidental noise, a very common situation outside laboratory conditions. The approach presented in the last section constitutes a possible solution to this problem.

Faced with these difficulties, pattern recognition may take advantage of "high-level" linguistic knowledge concerning the structure (syntax) and meaning (semantics) of input messages. The interpretation of input signals is also necessary in order for the machine to perform an "intelligent" interaction with its human partner (Sabbah, 1989). Pragmatic knowledge linked with both the task in hand and the current user's model may also help solve the misunderstandings often encountered with natural spoken language (Matrouf, 1990; Luzzati, 1991).

Considering all these requirements, a huge amount of information must be supported by a human-machine communication systems dealing with a natural, continuous and linguistic input. Knowledge may be organised into a hierarchy of more or less abstract levels, from *signal features* to *scripts* and *goals*, corresponding to a vertical organisation of the whole set of internal representations. In the case of multi-modality, the situation seems even more complex, since a horizontal organisation corresponding to several parallel modalities or analyses is mixed with the vertical one. Even further, if messages generated by the machine remain under its control through a feedback loop, in a human-like way, this means that perceptual procedures must check the validity of production on-line, and thus work simultaneously with generation procedures. This high degree of parallelism and real-time processing calls for an adapted machine architecture, in which any piece of information may instantaneously contribute to the whole process.

Multi-modality in human-machine communications

The combination of several modalities may improve human-machine interactions, for the benefit of both perceptual (machine input) and production (machine output) aspects. If efficient natural language interpretation and production devices were involved, a multi-modal system would become more natural, allowing human-like interactions. This is of course the ultimate goal of research in human-machine communication, and also the goal fixed by Artificial Intelligence: to design a machine that would behave like a human being in a dialogue situation.

The following properties can provide solutions to problems outlined previously, for the interpretation of a message, learning and production aspects.

- *Interpretation of user messages by the machine*

Each modality may be specialized in a certain type of input. Thus, the number of messages that can possibly be treated by a given modality is restricted, which goes towards reducing ambiguity.

A typical example of this processing architecture may be found in an elementary graphical edition task, which combines speech recognition and a computer mouse (Bolt, 1980). Speech conveys simple commands, the parameters of which are entered with a mouse. Our architect's apprentice may for instance ask the system to change the location of a piece of furniture through the elementary command: "Put that there" (or "Put that here") and click the mouse twice. The first click must roughly coincide with the pronunciation of the word "that", and indicate the location of an object. The second click occurs at the same time as the word "there", and shows the destination of the object. If no modality other than speech were available, the message would be somewhat more difficult to understand (i.e.: "take the big cupboard which is in the room at the top of the screen, to the left of the washing room, and put it in the dining-room, about twenty-two centimetres to the right of the TV").

Instead of being specialized, modalities could potentially replace each other, depending on the user's preference, environmental context and current state of activity in communication channels. A given modality, say a two-dimensional gesture, can be expressed through a choice of channels, for instance a tactile screen or mouse. The system environment may impose strong constraints on the modality to be chosen. Although speech can be used by aircraft pilots to make inquiries to the control system about the plane situation, it must be replaced by another modality when speed increases (Barès et al., 1991; Perbet et al., 1991).

Following a different processing strategy, several modalities may simultaneously participate in the analysis of several dimensions of the same message. Results of complementary analyses may be associated to recognize any input through fusion. For instance, a user's utterance may be processed by a speech recogniser, while lip movements are read by a visual analyser (Robert-Ribes, 1992; Brooke, 1991). This association of correlated acoustic and visual signals may particularly facilitate the recognition of speech affected by noise.

- *Machine message production*

Conversely, when the machine produces speech sounds, it may display a face drawn on the screen, whose lips move consistently with the acoustic signal (Benoit, 1991). From a more general point of view, the specialized and parallel nature of perceptual modalities may also characterise the part of the machine aimed at generating messages. Specialization may help the user to guess the topic of a message, if each output modality is associated with a certain type of information. For instance, assuming a multiple voice stereo synthesiser, error messages could be simulated as if coming from a specific spatial location, and conveyed by a gloomy male voice, whereas running dialogue sentences could use a soft female voice coming apparently from another source.

Local variations of brightness or colour would catch the user's eye on a particular object on the screen, and could be used in parallel with the synthesiser. Coming back to our preliminary imaginary scenario, the machine may visually indicate a missing component in the house plan, display its written form, while telling the novice why it must be included in the architecture. The equivalence of several modalities for expressing the same idea is essential for a visually impaired user. A braille display and speech synthesiser may together improve the lucidity of the message (Burger, 1992). Thus, several output modalities may be specialized and cooperate with each other, in the same way as input modalities.

In order to approximate human behaviour, cross relationships between perception and production should also be considered (Burnod, 1989).

Fast decisions concerning actions to be triggered and the way to continue those already begun may be based on current perceptions. An example of user's movement perception may be found in simulations of virtual worlds (Krueger, 1990). Perceiving the environment as well as its own actions would provide the machine with an accurate means of communication. Then, detecting a hesitation of the user could be interpreted as a sign of misunderstanding, and result in a different formulation or turning to another modality. When synthesisers are close to human vocal ability, their prosodic parameters will possibly be adapted on-line to changes of situation. As we proceed, multi-modality appears not only as a gadget intended to improve human-computer interactions, but also as a compelled pathway to more sophisticated machines, with human skills.

- *Machine learning*

Learning holds a prime position among human skills. But not all modalities are learned completely individually: learning to use our vocal tract so as to pronounce words is partly controlled by hearing; and learning to read relies on vision, audition and speech production. Within an artificial system, the acquisition of a representation in a new modality could refer to other dimensions of the event, already known by different modalities.

The system should be able to self-adaptation to situations that have inevitably not been forecasted by its designers. This requires a learning procedure which may be triggered at any time, in a certain context. Such contextual, "never-ending" learning is proposed in the last section of this article. It may be noticed that holding a dialogue requires keeping track of peculiarities which means that the system must adapt during the course of processing. Natural language interactions usually provide the opportunity to exchange information.

If a multi-modal system was able to integrate efficient analysers and action generation devices, the latter would benefit from simultaneous perception in order to learn new actions. Only efficient actions would be retained among a set of randomly generated ones. In this case, multimodality appears to be the most natural way of dealing with action learning.

A STATE OF THE ART

Only recently has multi-modality really appeared in the field of Human-Machine Communication (Bolt, 1980). Consequently, the part played in research topics such as ergonomics, speech processing, vision, system architecture and tools is not yet fixed, neither are specific technical terms. These questions are still being dealt with (Coutaz, 1991; IHM-M'92, 1992; Bellik & Teil, 1992(a)).

However, one can consider that a multi-modal human-machine communication system is characterised by the automatic extraction of the meaning of the expressions it manipulates. It can extract the meaning of an interaction built up from several modalities. In monomodal human-machine communication expressions are divided into elementary messages. In multi-modality, these messages can be conveyed by several modalities. During generation, a multi-modal system can select several output modalities and generate information about these modalities.

Types of multi-modality

Several types of multi-modality, concerning both perception and generation, may be distinguished in current investigations. The following figures summarize the classification proposed by Bellik & Teil (1992a), and illustrate it by examples involving two perceptual devices: a speech recogniser and a mouse driver. A complete multi-modal system should make it possible to enter any of these modes.

The user and the machine have to know at all times:
• which type of multi-modality can be used next,
• which type of multi-modality is currently being used by the other (in particular, it is necessary to know if simultaneous messages are independent so that fusion must not occur).

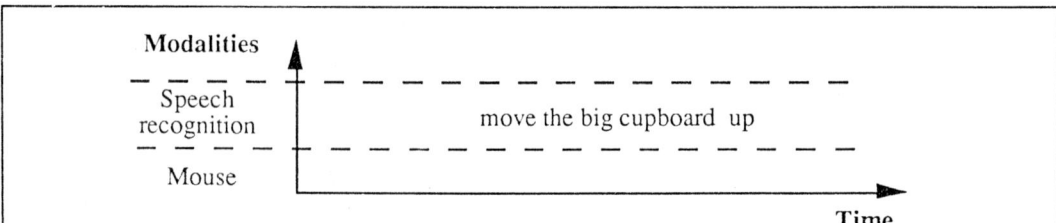

Fig. 1. a. Exclusive multi-modality.

Each expression is produced in turn using only one modality (a single modality is used at any one time). This type of multi-modality only allows the choice of the modality on which an expression will be conveyed. The choice can be made according to the user, environment, current state of the modalities... In the example above, the user transmitted the whole expression "move the big cupboard up" solely with the speech recognition channel.

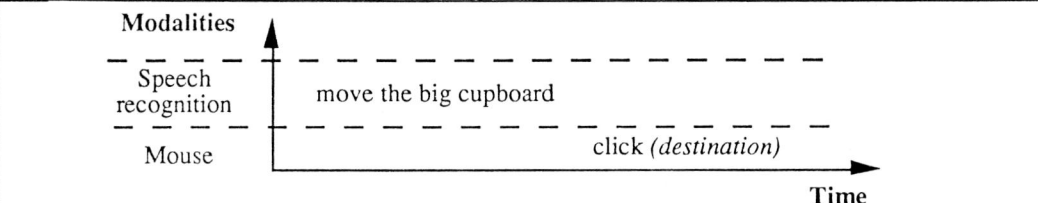

Fig. 1. b. Alternate multi-modality.

Each expression is produced in turn, and use of several modalities but only one at a time. This type of multi-modality allows the division of an expression into several messages, each being transmitted through the most appropriate modality. In the above example, it is difficult for the user to utter the precise destination of the object without the mouse. The meaning to be associated with the mouse click is written in italics. But with this type of multi-modality, the interpretation of a message depends on the syntax in a rather static way (in the example above, after an object has been selected, the system will interpret the next click as a destination).

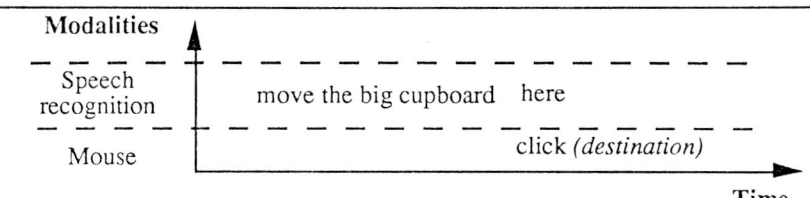

Fig. 1. c. Synergic multi-modality.

Each expression is produced in turn, and can make use of several modalities at a time. In this type of multi-modality, the meaning to be associated with a message can be conveyed by another message in a different modality. Messages associated with the same meaning must trigger a fusion process. Several criteria can be considered (temporal proximity between "here" and "click" in this example). Speech recognition can use a multi-modal context (mouse event detection) to facilitate the recognition of specific words (here, there...).

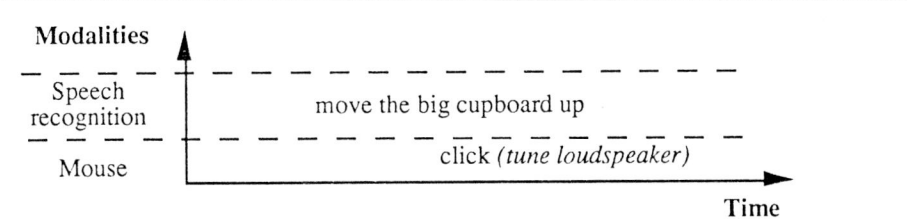

Fig. 1. d. Concurrent multi-modality.

Since several modalities can be used at a given time, the user or the machine can send independent messages simultaneously on different modalities. Simultaneous messages from independent expressions must not be merged. In the example above, the user wants to move an object and, at the same time, to adjust the loudspeaker level. The interpretation of the vocal expression "move the big cupboard up" must be made independently of the interpretation of the mouse click on the slide button regulating the output level of the loudspeaker.

Implementing multi-modality

The multi-modal perspective is quite attractive, especially when considering the possibility that we could, one day, hold a conversation with a machine with no more constraints than with a human partner. But this will be at the expense of deep effort in integrating and controlling many communication channels within the same system. Facing this challenge, we may question current machine architectures. But most researchers are currently working towards a less ambitious goal, which is to bring together communication channels of moderate ability in order for them to support each other. Deficiencies in current pattern recognition systems may thus be compensated for by other input channels. Given the slow rate of possible interactions between modalities in current implementations, serial architectures still suffice.

Although it may solve some difficulties encountered by current communication devices, multi-modality poses its own set of problems. Temporal distortions not only impede the recognition of a single pattern, but also the time relation between modalities. Different messages conveyed in parallel by several input channels, and participating in the same task, must be adequately united in accordance with a number of factors: knowledge about current dialogue state, characteristics of input modalities. The following criteria may be combined: a priori semantic relationships between modalities, temporal and spatial relationships, constraints concerning possible or forbidden combinations... A single criterion is often inadequate to unite messages. With regard to concurrent multi-modality (Fig. 1.d.), the sole detection of time coincidence has a good chance of uniting input streams that should be considered independent. But temporal relations between channels must be detected and created, to simulate cooperation between channels, such as substitution, complementarity, multi-modal learning. Returning to our prototypical example: "Put that there" combined with mouse clicks is the coincidence of messages from two modalities, together with syntactic information which allow the system to understand its input signals. Assuming that a given concept is referred to by a word already known by the machine acoustic channel. The simultaneous auditory and graphical presentation of this concept may then help in the learning of the visual representation. Here again, the management of parallel flows of data appears to be of prime necessity.

Both Natural Language Generation (Dale et al., 1990) and image synthesis are under study, mostly independently. As a matter of fact, multi-modal generation has not yet been investigated extensively. We consider that the parallel generation of messages through several channels requires a parallel and highly interactive architecture, in particular if generation can permanently be controlled by perceptual modalities. Before proposing such a computational architecture, we present a selection of existing multi-modal systems.

Description of some multi-modal systems

Several multi-modal systems have already been implemented and aim at solving some of the problems listed in the previous section. Each of the following illustrative systems can be described by: the set of modalities, domain of application, types of multi-modality, software architecture, knowledge representation, mechanisms used for fusion.

(1) "Put That There", MIT (Bolt, 1980).

(2) CUBRICON, (Neal, 1988).

(3) Gerbal, Boeing (Salisbury et al. 1990).

(4) The SHIVA workstation (Bellik & Teil, 1992(b); Teil & Bellik, 1991).

(5) ICP/DRAW, ICP (Caelen, 1991).

(6) MMI2, ESPRIT Project (Wilson, 1991).

(7) DRET, LIMSI and Sextant Avionique (Barès et al., 1992; Perbet et al., 1991).

(8) MELODIA, Thomson and CRIN/INRIA (Nogier, 1992).

(9) LOIR, IRIT, (Azémard et al., 1992).

- *Same set of modalities and applications*

Most systems use speech recognition, speech synthesis, designation with a mouse, graphic display. They are applied to graphical editors (1, 4, 5, 6), air traffic control (2, 3, 8), pilot assistance (7).

- *Multi-modal knowledge*

Besides classical knowledge bases found in monomodal dialogue handlers, specific multi-modal knowledge is involved (Caelen, 1991(a)). For instance, the description of the possible combinations or incompatibilities between modalities can be formalised in a declarative way with rules. In perception, such rules drive the recognition and the interpretation of the multi-modal messages, taking into account the multi-modal context. For instance,
IF (*mouse event has been detected* AND *word "put" has already been recognised*)
THEN (*facilitate the recognition of "that", "here"...*)

In generation, such rules select the output modalities and the messages to be produced:
IF (*user is currently speaking*)
THEN (*do not use speech synthesiser*)

In (7), a multi-modal grammar is composed of rules which drive recognition or generation. In (9), the interpretation consists in building conceptual graphs with the help of such rules.

- *Modular functional architectures*

The functional architecture is composed of several levels (input and output, dialogue, application). Thus the same system is supposed to be used easily with other modalities or other applications. At each of these functional levels, the knowledge is divided between several interacting modules (see for instance, figure 2).

Each of these modules contains knowledge such as the language used in this modality (lexical, syntaxical, semantic informations) or one kind of knowledge usual in monomodal systems (model of the application, model of the user, model of the system, current state of the application, current state of the user, current state of the system, dialogue history).

For instance, three functional levels (input/output, dialogue, application) contain expert modules in (6). An expert module performs a specific task (dialogue context expert, user modelling expert...) or deals with a specific modality (natural language experts, graphics and gesture experts). The dialogue controller handles the dialogue and activates whatever experts are necessary to support dialogue function.

In (7), knowledge is divided into several layers which contain the state of different tasks that can be performed by the pilot, the commands which can be used to change the state of a task, the different ways (channels, modalities) of carrying out each task, a multi-modal grammar.

- *Symbolic representation of knowledge*

The representation of knowledge in these modules is symbolic. Data are represented in an explicit and often structured way. Multi-modal integration seldom appears at the signal level.

- *Predominance of temporal proximity criterion for fusion*

Fusion of multi-modal messages depends mainly on temporal proximity and syntaxical or semantic knowledge. In the "put that there" example, the user never clicks on the object to be moved and utters "that" exactly at the same time. Variability is supported by the use of a temporal window. Events detected in the same temporal window are considered to be correlated.

- Integration of heterogeneous systems

For instance speech and gestures are first analysed individually into symbolic representations (sequence of words for speech) before fusion of both modalities. The analysis made in each modality often uses modality-specific representations, existing software and/or hardware. The multi-modal system aims at the integration of these heterogeneous modality-specific systems. The multi-modal system has to take into account the different durations of recognition or production in each modality-specific system.

For instance, in (4) the low level events issued from each media are dated and translated into higher level information by an interpreter and a language model associated with this medium. This high-level information is inserted into a waiting list which follows the corresponding event chronology. A manager analyses the waiting list with the help of a model of the application (commands and corresponding list of arguments).

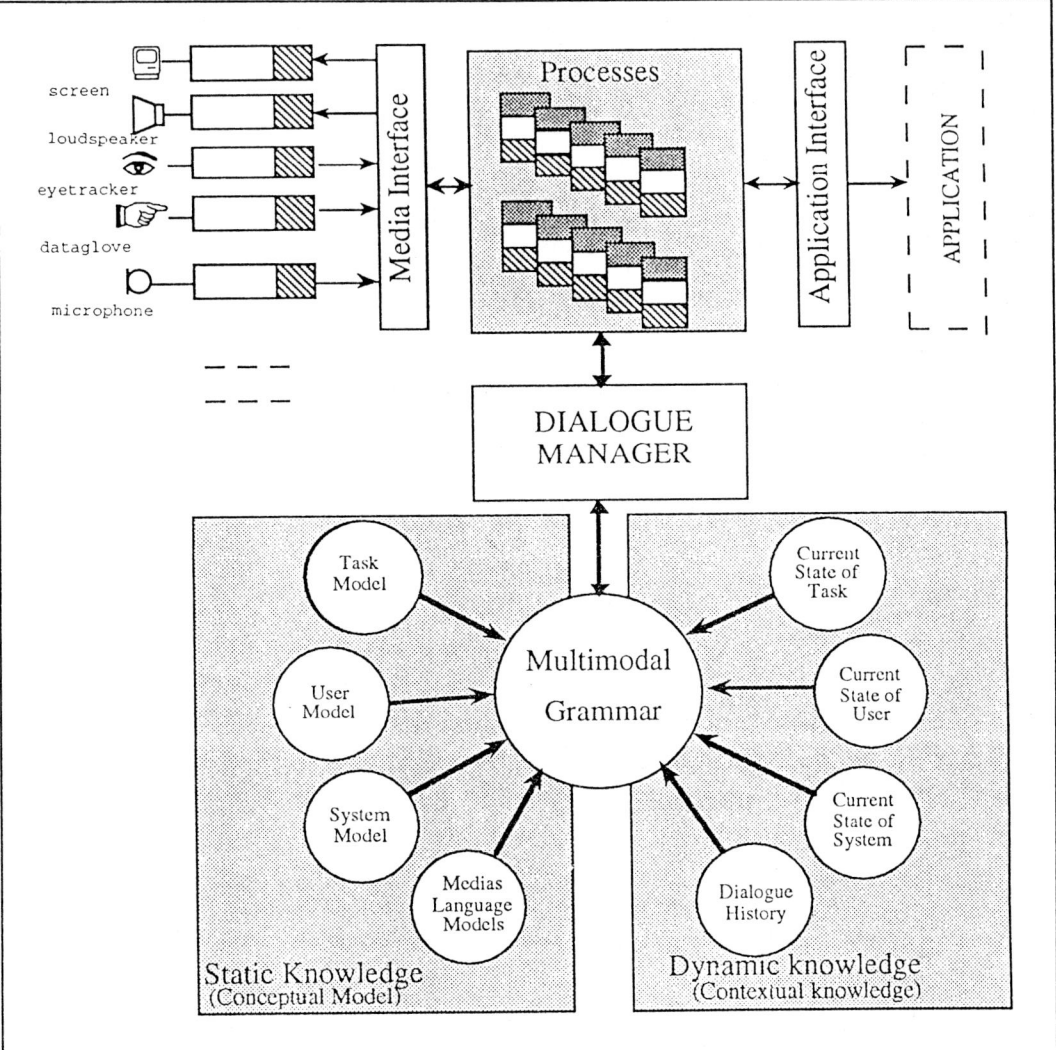

Fig. 2. by K. Matrouf, cf (Barès et al., 1991).
The dialogue manager triggers actions (called processes). Processes are selected with rules of the multi-modal grammar. This grammar incorporates several modules of knowledge.

- *Modality specific data are translated into a common formalisms*

Knowledge is represented and transmitted between modalities or modules using a common formalism, which facilitates:
- the substitution of a non available modality by another (the common formalism is used as a pivot),
- the transfer of knowledge between modalities (representations of knowledge in one modality can be translated into another modality through this common formalism),

- the rapid integration of messages perceived in several modalities (once modality-specific messages are translated in this common formalism, multi-modal integration is supposedly easier),
- the reusability of other modalities or applications (when a new modality is incorporated, it only needs the procedures translating its specific formalism into the common formalism).

For instance, in (6), all the messages exchanged between modules follow the same language of semantic representation (Common Meaning Representation).

- *Use of contextual information*

Contextual information concerning the state of the task, events detected in the different modalities, dialogue history... is used to merge multi-modal data and solve ambiguity. In (3), operational context, graphical events (designation of objects or locations) are used to disambiguate speech input (facilitation of compatible speech input).

- *Specific interesting features of multi-modality*

In (2), when an object is selected by the machine, it is indicated to the user through the combination of speech synthesisers and graphical displays. This semantic redundancy and modality complementarity facilitate the perception of the selected object by the user. Specific functions can be accessed via specific modalities. In the air traffic control application presented in (8), the operator can manipulate three-dimensional representations of the traffic with a dataglove.

Other presentations of multi-modal systems may be found in Wilson & Conway 1991; Coutaz, 1992; IHM'92/IMAL; Bourguet, 1992.

TOWARDS A MULTI-MODAL MACHINE BASED ON COINCIDENCE DETECTION

The requirements of a multi-modal system may be summarised by a few points, ordered according to priority:
- Real-time co-ordination of communication channels based on both environmental features and internal knowledge; in particular, the generation part should be context-dependent, that is influenced in the course of its accomplishment by environmental signals, including the perception of the resulting action itself.
- Even if partly compensated by the presence of multiple potential means of communication, factors such as variability and noise that affect recognition should be considered in each modality. Variability of the generation part (choice of an output channel, speech prosody) may be implemented, in order to make it more efficient and less tiresome.
- Adaptive skill should be as autonomous as possible, not limited to a preliminary "learning phase", involving reliable knowledge previously acquired in other modalities.

A real-time processing principle

Homogeneity of the system representations and processes is a minimal requirement for avoiding response time delays.

Assuming that all pieces of knowledge must talk to each other in order to understand input messages, it would be better if they were not disturbed by language problems. Any translation costs time. This is the reason why, in the memory model presented here, the same kind of internal representation for pattern recognition as well as for symbolic processing and pattern generation is used (Béroule, 1985, 1992).

A basic piece of data which mainly inspired this memory model is taken from neurobiology, and concerns the way neurons integrate their input: the more synchronized the signals activating a neuron, the faster its response. This may be interpreted as coding information by considering significant the time at which any signal reaches a certain location in memory, relative to other signals. Brain circuitry might involve coincidence detectors for this purpose. It may be noticed that this temporal coding has never been used in computational architectures, for it needs an accurate timing of internal data flows. It is easier to store data inside a passive permanent memory, without caring about the exact time at which it will be subsequently used. Whatever the congestion of data traffic in the machine, the value contained in a register and its relative location in memory are significant, not the time at which the register is accessed. Not only Von Neumann conventional computers are concerned, but also parallel architectures. In synchronous systems involving a matrix of microprocessors, such as systolic architectures, access time is tied to a central clock, the same for each processor. Time cannot be a discriminant dimension. A more recent, non synchronous system allows a dynamic virtual configuration of processors (*Connexion Machine*); but the route taken by messages towards a certain processor depends on the variable traffic on data buses, and so is the transfer time.

Previously put forward as a requirement of multi-modality, coincidence detection could form the basic principle of a complete system, provided that its own constraints be satisfied. This means that human-machine communication problems should be approached from a slightly different point of view. First of all, understanding a user's message is performed through matching it with internal representations of the machine. In classical architectures, this is performed through register-to-register comparisons. An equivalent functionality is to be found with coincidence detection...

Since coincidence detection is carried out between internal signals, some of them may be associated with an unknown input pattern, whereas other signals may stand for the system's internal representations. The "best match" between input and references will correspond to the best coincidence between associated signals. This alternative procedure can be implemented by intersecting pathways which convey internal "knowledge" signals with pathways which carry input signals. Elementary processors (or cells) detect possible temporal and spatial matching at each point of intersection, and generate an internal signal proportional to the level of coincidence. Cells can be chained along a pathway according to the time organisation of series of inputs; this means that the first cell will be associated with events by which an input begins, the second cell will be fed by the following events, and so on until the last cell of the pathway receives the last events. The final level of activity of a given pathway will then depend on the serial contribution of its cells (Fig. 3). This space-time integration of input is referred to as Guided Propagation, since the internal flow of signals is guided by inputs towards characteristic memory locations, situated at the end of internal pathways.

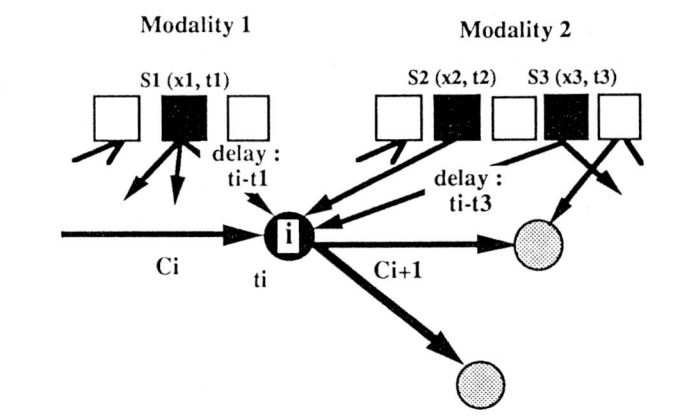

Fig. 3. Multi-modal integration with coincidence detection.
One of the context dependent cells (circles), CD_i, is fully activated (in black) by the coincidence of a contextual signal C_i and stimuli S_j characterised by their space-time location (x_j, t_j) occupied by detectors (squares). The threshold of cell i determines the logic function computed by the cell ("OR", "AND"...). The activation produced by cell i propagates as a contextual signal C_{i+1} towards two other cells which may later receive incoming stimulations. When context cells are linked to detectors, delays are computed so that signals sent by detectors reach the context cell at the same time. In the example given above, detectors S_j are activated at different times t_j, CD_i at time t_i, thus the delays of links S_j -CD_i are set to t_i-t_j.

Guided Propagation is inherently real-time. Coincidence detection of signals is performed instantaneously, contrary to the comparison of complex messages. Furthermore, signals taking the shape of activation levels are easier to generate than complex messages. The main reason why the global response-time does not increase with the amount of internal representations or possible input may be explained if noticing that there are as many cells as possible contexts for any given input item. When this item occurs, the input flow propagates towards each "Context-dependent" cell. If it coincides somewhere with an internal flow, the item has found an interpretation; the memory subset activated by the input has got an intersection with the subset activated by the internal "expectation" flow. Since activation spreads in parallel in different directions, the duration of this "set intersection search" does not depend on the size of the memory subset under consideration, which correspond to the current amount of knowledge.

Multiple modules for multi-modality

Internal representations of continuous environmental signals are formed of discrete space-time locations. In other words, the activation at a certain time of an event-detector located in memory at a certain space position means that its associated event has been identified. A keyboard input is perfectly adapted to this way of coding. A source of difficulty comes from the necessary transformation of complex continuous signals propagating in the environment, into discrete space-time events, which form the single representation that can be treated by our memory model.

It has been demonstrated that speech could be adequately represented by a distribution of spectral events. Input to the speech recogniser is formed by a bank of feature-detectors which are activated according to the distribution of spectral events: a spectrogram resembles a musical score, with its discrete signs distributed in time and pitch (frequency) dimension. This analogy may illustrate the robustness of this representation to superimposed sounds. When voices are mixed, a situation commonly encountered in cocktail parties, our representation contains events corresponding to each voice and which can cohabit in the same spectrum, similar to notes representing several instruments which cohabit in a full score.

The automatic recognition of a given space-time distribution of discrete events corresponding for instance to a word is characterised by the activation of a specific word-detector situated at the end of a memory pathway. The part played by a bank of such word-detectors can be very similar to that of feature-detectors, that is to guide propagation along deeper pathways which represent semantic or syntactic associations of words. Pathways that code the same characteristic are grouped within the same module, and the set of modules is organised following the vertical and horizontal setting outlined previously (Fig. 6).

Pattern recognition is obviously not the whole story. A multi-modal system must be able to take decisions, favour an appropriate selection of modalities in a certain context, and generate patterns. This is possible in this architecture in which autonomous internal representations can be activated without incoming stimulations, thanks to high-level decisions. A script module may facilitate propagation in certain perceptual modules, check the result of recognition and then activate a couple of syntactic and semantic structures to generate a speech output. From a technical point of view, *facilitation* is implemented by a wave of threshold reduction which proceeds in the opposite direction to activation. Amazingly, both activation and facilitation are used in each module. In perceptual modules, the activation flow is prevalent but chooses preferably facilitated pathways. In production modules, heavy facilitation is regulated by "proprioceptive" activation. In this parallel architecture, each module may work at the same time, allowing production modules to be controlled on-line thanks to perceptual information.

A Control Unit is aimed at checking the whole architecture function and exerts in return its influence, only through the modulation of cell parameters. The creation of new memory pathways in the course of processing (*dynamic learning*), which is a main feature of the approach, requires cell parameters to be set in a particular configuration. This regulation is carried out by the central controller, possibly towards a single module while the other modules still work in the "recognition" mode. These latter modules identify one aspect of the currently learned pattern, and may facilitate selectively the corresponding pathway in the module currently being learned.

Other parameters, in particular temporal ones (*time-delays*) can be modified by the Control Unit, which may change the rhythm of a sentence during its generation. The balance between internal and incoming flows of signals can be changed so as to temporarily favour stimuli (*data-driven* mode) or the system's expectations (*knowledge-driven* mode). The result of a recognition task in parallel modalities is checked by the controller, by considering the amount of activated detectors at the output of every module.

An ambiguous pattern will induce the activation of more than one detector, whereas an unknown pattern is characterised by a lack of activation which would trigger a learning phase.

The parallel nature of modulation procedures does not impede the speed of the system, contrary to a serial computer control unit. Its future development may benefit from research in neurobiology devoted to neuromodulation (Tassin, 1992).

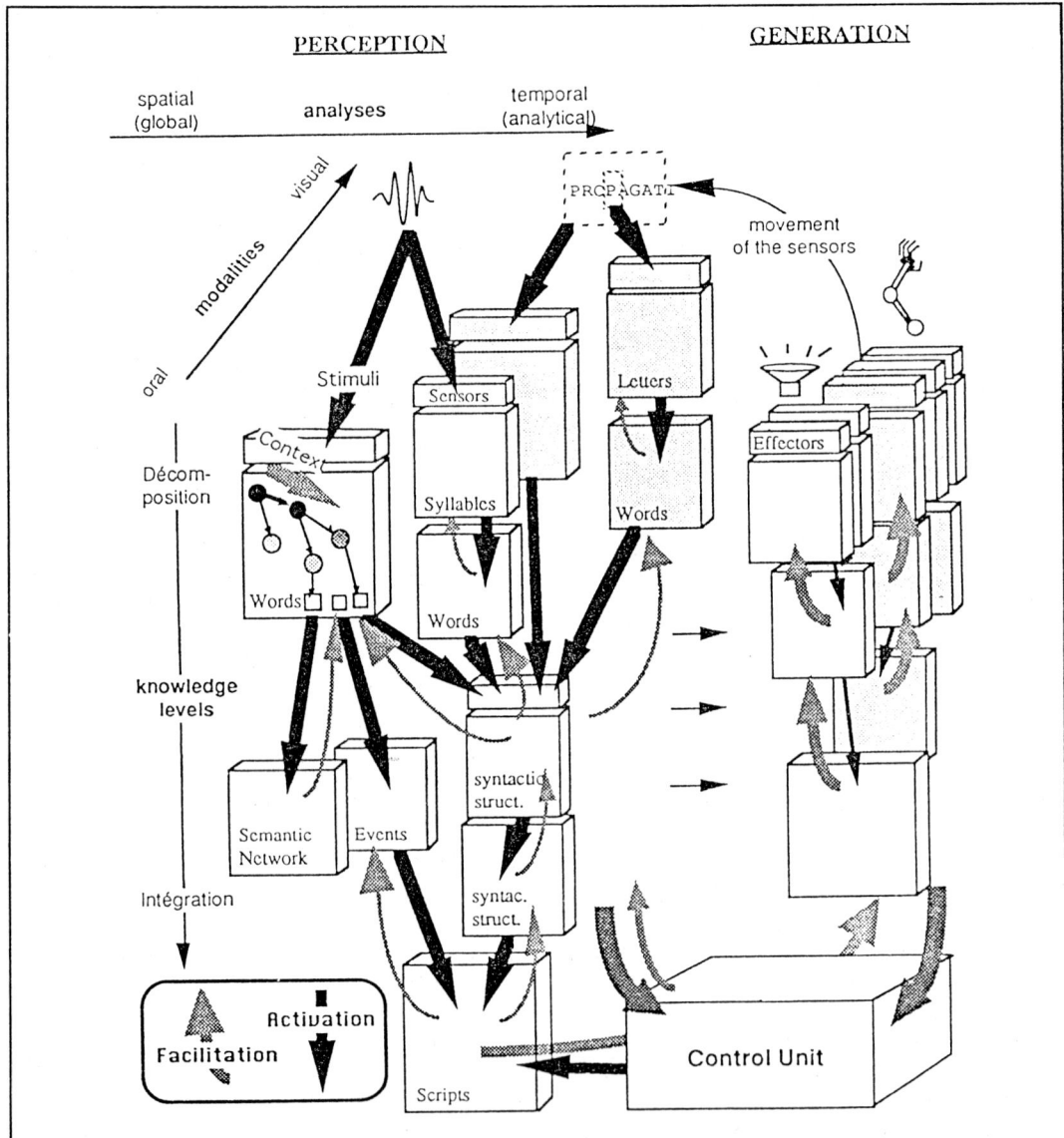

Fig. 6. Planned human-machine communication system, based on Guided Propagation (detection of coincidence between Contextual signals and Stimuli). The parameters of elementary cells are modulated by a Control Unit. The activation flow is predominant in perception modules, whereas facilitation is mainly used in generation modules.

Current simulations

Guided Propagation Networks have been applied to separate tasks involved in human-machine communication: speech recognition, syntactic learning, semantic processing, adaptive scanning of visual words, generation of action. The integration of several modules in the same system is under way (Fig. 4, 5). An experiment of question/answering has been carried out, which involves four modules respectively responsible for semantic inferences, dialogue history, scripts and sentence generation. An interesting point is the cooperation between modules working in the same layer. The input composed of a set of word-detectors can activate the semantic network, which then facilitates inferred words, which activate statements contained in the dialogue history. Thus, statements concerned by a user question can be retrieved, thanks to semantic inferences.

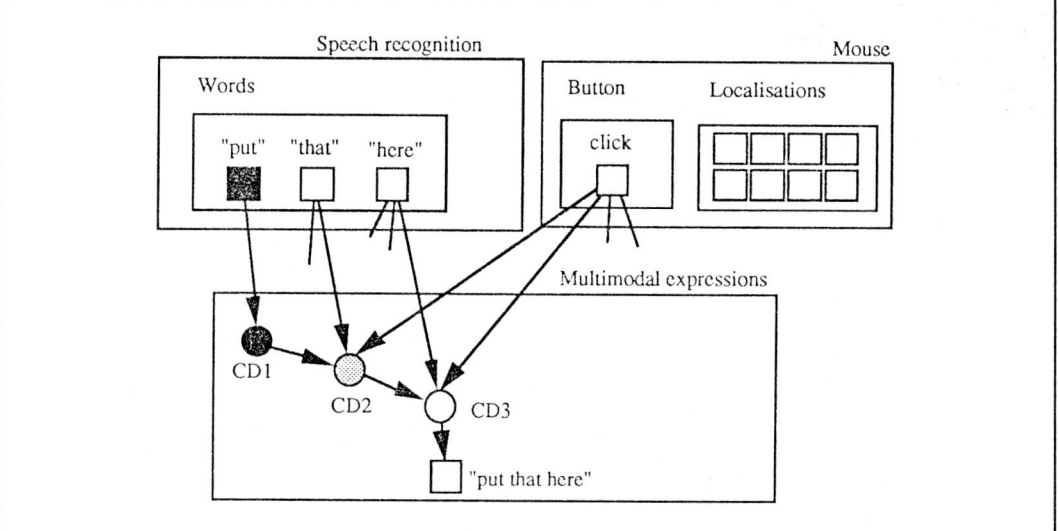

Fig. 4. Syntaxical representation of a multi-modal command.
Each modality is represented by a module which contains detectors corresponding to events perceived in this modality. A module "Multi-modal expressions" detects combinations of sequences and coincidences between signals sent by detectors. It therefore uses Context Dependent (CD) cells. For instance, the recognition of the word "put" induces the activation of the detector associated with this word; this sends a signal to the context cell CD1 which becomes activated; CD1 sends a contextual signal to CD2 which means that the beginning of the command "put that here" has been recognized; CD2 will be fully activated if the word "that" and a mouse click are then recognized ...

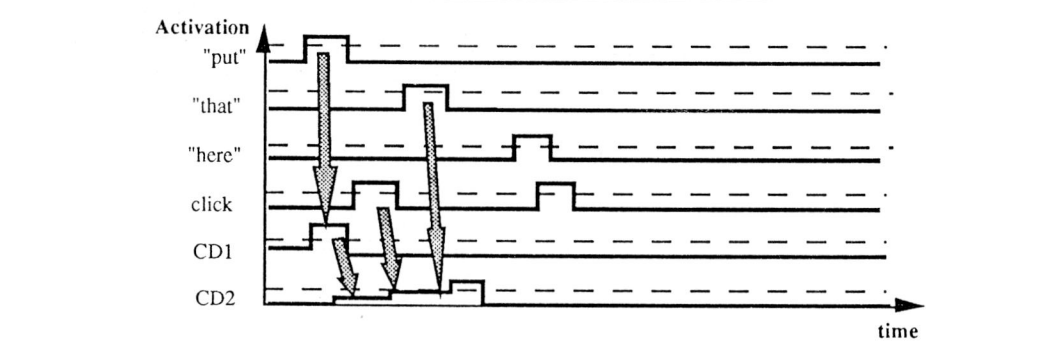

Fig. 5. Activity histogram of cells in figure 4 during the recognition of the multi-modal command "put that here". The activation (bold line) of each cell depends on its input signals. If this value increases above the cell's threshold (dotted line), then the cell produces a signal and sends it to its output cells. In the example given above, CD2 receives successively a contextual signal sent by CD1 which means that the word "put" has been recognized, a signal sent by the cell associated with the mouse click, and a signal sent by the cell associated with the word "that". These three signals last a certain time, so that they do not need to arrive exactly at the same time and in the same order to activate CD2.

In such a hard-wired architecture, a major problem concerns the representation of variables. The henceforward famous phrase "put that there" contains two variables: a variable object (that) and a variable location (there). Obviously, not all possible combinations of object and locations can be reasonably represented by as many memory pathways. This problem has, uptil now, received two possible solutions. Considering the dynamic nature of pathways, variables can be considered as temporary cells. Solving a problem then requires the creation of many pathways corresponding to hypothetical combinations for getting closer to a known goal (Blanchet, 1992). Another solution involves the precise time coding of signals, in accordance with a neurobiological phenomenon called synchrony (Frégnac, 1991). In this perspective, the cell corresponding to a variable and the cell corresponding to its value would both generate synchronized signals. This dynamic assignment of variables through this temporal phase association mechanism is presently under study in the framework of multimodality (Martin, 1993).

CONCLUSION

The distance left before being able to design a machine similar to the fictionary one described in the introduction of this paper can now be evaluated. Among the set of possible modalities involving continuous signals, speech and vision have an opposing status. Whereas speech can now be recognised with reasonable accuracy, except in the presence of accidental noise, computer vision has not yet reached the same level of efficiency. Visual and acoustic output can be roughly linked with variations in the environment so as to simulate a virtual world, but text-to-speech synthesis is still produced out of context, without a perceptual feedback loop: current systems do not listen to their own utterances.

At the level of message interpretation, Natural Language constitutes a major topic of Artificial Intelligence, but spontaneous vocal language is very rarely investigated, with its range of hesitations, noise, misconstructions and strange expressions. Future generations of multi-modal systems would benefit from the necessary improvement of each of these perception, language processing and production devices. In our opinion, in particular for satisfying the real-time constraint, these devices should preferably be developed within the same computational framework.

As a final remark, it may be noticed that multi-modality is rooted in different research fields such as Computer Science (multi-medias and multi-modal systems; audio-tactile images; direct manipulation of data), Psychology (modality-specific and multimodal mental representations; scene analysis and psycholinguistics) and Neurobiology (visual, auditory, somato-sensory and associative cortical areas; fusion and segregation of several analyses of visual stimuli). No doubt that the fusion of the respective contributions of these disciplines would be of great benefit to each of them.

REFERENCES

Azémard F., Macchion J.P. & Mieulet F. (1992), Multimodal: le réflexe pour une stratégie d'interprétation, *Quatrièmes journées sur l'ingénierie des interfaces homme-machine (IHM'92), 30/11/92-2/12/92*, Paris.

Barès M. & Néel F., Teil D. & Martin J.-C. (1992), Organisation d'une démarche conceptuelle pour modéliser l'interaction homme-machine: application au copilote électronique,. *Actes du colloque "L'interface des mondes réels et virtuels" organisé par EC2.*, 23-27 Mars 1992.

Bellik Y. & Teil D. (1992 (a)), Les types de multimodalité, *Quatrièmes journées sur l'ingénierie des interfaces homme-machine (IHM'92), 30/11/92-2/12/92*, Paris.

Bellik Y. & Teil D. (1992(b)), Multimodal Dialogue Interface, *WWDU'92*, Berlin, 1-4 Sept. 1992.

Benoit C. (1991), A promising challenge for bimodal machine-man communication. Taylor M.M., Néel F. Bouwhuis D.G. (eds), In *Proceedings of the Second Venaco Workshop on the Structure of Multimodal Dialogue*, Italy, Sept 16-20, 1991.

Béroule D., (1985), Un modèle de mémoire adaptative dynamique et associative pour le traitement automatique de la parole, *Thèse 3ème cycle, Orsay.* Mai 1985.

Béroule D. (1992), *Représentation Topologique Spatio-Temporelle pour la Communication Homme-Machine, Cognition, Perception, et Action dans la Communication Parlée*, J. Caelen, J.-L. Schwartz, C. Abry (Eds), Presses Universitaires de France, Paris.

Blanchet P. (1992), Une architecture connexionniste pour l'apprentissage par l'expérience et la représentation des connaissances, *Thèse 3ème cycle, Orsay.* Décembre 1992.

Bolt R. (1980), *Put That There: Voice and Gesture at the Graphics Interface*, Tech. report. MIT, Cambridge, Mass, 1980.

Bourguet M.L. (1992), Conception et réalisation d'une interface de dialogue personne-machine multimodale, *Thèse, INPG*, 27 Nov 1992.

Bradffort A., Baudel T. & Teil, D. (1992), Utilisation des gestes de la main pour l'interaction homme-machine, *Quatrièmes journées sur l'ingénierie des interfaces homme-machine (IHM'92)*, 30/11/92-2/12/92, Paris.

Brooke N.M., (1991), Processing facial images to enhance speech communication, Taylor M.M., Néel F. Bouwhuis D.G. (eds), In *Proceedings of the Second Venaco Workshop on the Structure of Multimodal Dialogue*, Italy, Sept 16-20, 1991.

Burger D., (1992), La multimodalité: un moyen d'améliorer l'accessibilité des systèmes informatiques pour les personnes handicapées. L'exemple des interfaces non-visuelles,. *ERGO.IA 92*.

Burnod Y., (1989), *An adaptative neural network: the cerebral cortex*, Masson 1989.

Caelen J. (1991(a)), Interaction multimodale dans ICP draw: expérience et perspectives. *Actes PRC CHM Interaction multimodale*, Lyon, Avril 1991.

Caelen J., (1991(b)), Multimodal interaction: event management and experiments with ICP Draw. Taylor M.M., Néel F. Bouwhuis D.G. (1991), In *Proceedings of the Second Venaco Workshop on the Structure of Multimodal Dialogue*, Italy, Sept 16-20, 1991.

Calliope (1989), *La parole et son traitement automatique*, Masson.

Coutaz J., (1991), Multimodal et multimédia, *Actes PRC CHM Interaction multimodale*. Lyon, Avril 1991.

Coutaz J. (1992), Multimedia and Multimodal User Interfaces: A Software Engineering Perspective, *Submitted to the StPetersburg International Workshop on Human Computer Interaction*.

Dale R., Mellish C.& Zock M. (1990), *Current research in natural language generation*, Dale R., Mellish C., Zock M. (eds), Academic Press Limited, London.

Escande P. (1992), Reconnaissance de la parole par un modèle connexionniste à détection de coïncidences, *Thèse 3ème cycle.,Orsay*, Décembre 1992.

Frégnac Y. (1991), How many cycles make an oscillation, In *Representations of Vision: Trends and Tacit Assumptions*, Eds. Goréa A., Frégnac Y., Kapoula Z. & Finlay J. Cambridge University Press, p. 97-109.

Hartline P. (1985), Multimodal integration in the brain, Combining dissimilar views of the world. In *Comparative neurobiology: Modes of communication in the nervous system*, Ch 18. Ed Melvin J. Cohen. John Wiley & sons.

IHM'92/IMAL (1992), *Quatrièmes journées sur l'ingénierie des interfaces homme-machine, 30/11/92-2/12/92, Paris*, Compte rendu de l'atelier "Interfaces Multimodales et Architectures Logicielles". Participants à l'atelier: F. Azémard, T. Baudel, Y. Bellik, S-K. Bennacef, M-L. Bourguet, N. Carbonell, R. Caubet, J. Coutaz, V. Gaildrat, J-C. Martin, L. Nigay, K. Ouadou, P. Palanque, D. Teil, N. Vigouroux.

IHM-M'92, Compte-rendu du "workshop" IHM-M organisé par le GDR-PRC "communication homme-machine" à Dourdan les 13 & 14 Avril 1992, Caelen, J. *Actes des quatrièmes journées sur l'ingénierie des interfaces homme-machine*, 30/11/92-2/12/92, Paris.

Krueger M.W. (1990), *Artificial reality II*. Addison-Weysley.

Liénard J.-S. (1991), *Rapport C.O.S.T. Communication homme-machine*, Avril 1991.

Luzzati D. (1991), A dynamic dialog model for human machine communication. Taylor M.M., Néel F. Bouwhuis D.G. (eds), In *Proceedings of the Second Venaco Workshop on the Structure of Multimodal Dialogue*, Italy, Sept 16-20, 1991

Martin J.-C. (1993), Interaction Homme-Machine Multimodale et Neurobiologie de la Perception, *Colloque "Images et Langages: Multimodalité et Modélisation cognitive"*, Paris, 1er et 2 Avril 1993.

Martin J.-C. & Béroule D. (1992), Eléments de modélisation connexionniste pour l'interaction homme-machine multimodale, *IHM'92, Quatrièmes journées sur l'ingénierie des interfaces homme-machine*, 30/11/92-2/12/92, Paris.

Matrouf A.K. (1990), Un système de dialogue oral orienté par la tâche, *Thèse 3 ème cycle*, Orsay., Septembre 1990.

Neal J., Thielman C., Bettinger K. & Byoun, J. (1988), Multimodal references in human-computer dialogue, In *Proceedings of AAAI-88,*, p.819-823.

Nogier J.-F. (1992), Dialogue Multi-modal pour Systèmes de Contrôle & Surveillance. Ecole d'automne Thomson, *Man Machine Interaction, Jouy-en-Josas*, 7-11 Sept 1992.

Perbet J.N., Favot J.J. & Barbier, B. (1991), Interactive Display Concept for the next Generation Cockpit, Taylor M.M., Néel F. Bouwhuis D.G. (eds), In *Proceedings of the Second Venaco Workshop on the Structure of Multimodal Dialogue*, Italy, Sept 16-20, 1991.

Robert-Ribes J., Escudier P. & Schwartz J.-L. (1992), Intégration d'informations auditives et visuelles par réseaux de neurones artificiels pour la perception de voyelles dans le bruit, *Actes des 6èmes Journées Neurosciences et Sciences de l'Ingénieur (NSI)*, 25-28 Mai 1992, Oléron.

Roques R. & Béroule D. (1991), Strategies of unsupervised learning for a parallel parsing architecture, *IJCNN*, Seattle, Juillet 1991.

Sabah G. (1989), *L'intelligence artificielle et le langage*, Hermès, Paris.

Salisbury M.W., Hendrickson J.H., Lammers T.L., Fu C. & Moody, S.A. (1990), Talk and Draw: bundling speech and graphics, *IEEE Computer, 23(8)*, August, 1990, p.59-65.

Tassin J.P. (1992), Architectures et fonctions dans le Système Nerveux Central: l'importance des neuromodulateurs, *Actes NSI 1992*.

Teil D. & Bellik Y. (1991), Multimodal dialogue interface on a PC-like work station. Taylor M.M., Néel F. Bouwhuis D.G. (1991), In *Proceedings of the Second Venaco Workshop on the Structure of Multimodal Dialogue*, Italy, Sept 16-20, 1991.

Teil D., Da Silva O. (1991), Gesture recognition using a data glove input device. Taylor M.M., Néel F. Bouwhuis D.G. (1991), In *Proceedings of the Second Venaco Workshop on the Structure of Multimodal Dialogue*, Italy, Sept 16-20, 1991.

Wilson M.D. (1991), *The first MMI2 Demonstrator, Deliverable d7, Esprit Project 2474 MMI2, A Multi-Modal Interface for Man Machine interaction with Knowledge Based Systems*, Editor M.D. Wilson, July 1991.

Wilson M.D., Conway, A. (1991), Enhanced Interaction Styles for User Interfaces, *IEEE Computer Graphics and Applications*, vol 11, p.79-90.

Résumé

L'interaction homme-machine peut impliquer plusieurs canaux de communication en entrée et en sortie, organisé de façon à exhiber un comportement cohérent. On qualifie alors l'interaction de "multimodale". On montre que l'amélioration du naturel des interactions ainsi que d'autres avantages apportés par la multimodalité se soldent par des problèmes qui viennent s'ajouter à ceux rencontrés avec les systèmes monomodaux, comme par exemple la coordination en temps-réel des modalités, leur fusion, leur ségrégation et acquisition de compétence. Ces questions sont ensuite illustrées par une sélection de systèmes multimodaux. Une architecture de traitement temps-réel fondée sur la détection de coïncidences est enfin présentée comme une approche éventuelle du dialogue multimodal.

Access to Texts and Images

"Never imagine yourself not to be otherwise than what it might appear to others that what you were or might have been was not otherwise than what you had been would have appeared to them to be otherwise."

"I think I should understand that better", said Alice very politely, "if I had it written down."

Lewis Carroll

Tactile and audio-tactile images as vehicles for learning

Ronald A.L. Hinton

Tactile Diagrams Research Unit, Department of Education, Loughborough University of Technology, Loughborough, Leicestershire, LE11 3TU, United Kingdom

ABSTRACT

The information obtainable from a visual image is contrasted with that from a tactile image, and the limitations and ambiguities inherent in outline tactile drawings are pointed out. The use of textures and contrasts to minimise such problems is explained, and the importance of the memory component in tactual perception is emphasised. The needs of congenitally blind students are particulary discussed.

The new technology described includes the Nomad audio-tactile device and a variety of approaches to the design of a refreshable tactile graphics display from a number of researchers. Their present limitations as teaching resources, but future importance are mentioned.

THE IMPORTANCE OF TACTILE ILLUSTRATIONS

In modern education in most subjects and at all stages diagrams and pictures are an essential component and not just an embellishment Blind students need effective tactile alternatives to these and it is important that these alternatives keep pace with improvements in educational technology generally. As an educational researcher my major concern for the last seven years has been with the provision of clear and effective tactile illustrations of many kinds and with the perceptual and educational processes which enable these to be used by people with a severe visual impairment.

THE PERCEPTION OF VISUAL AND TACTILE PICTURES

The human hand is equipped to receive three-dimensional information about the three-dimensional world, and to make sensitive diagnoses from this information. Such information can include surface texture and assessments of movement, weight, and temperature, as well as details of gross shape.

With touch there is an obvious spatial correlation between the touch sensors and points on the boundaries of a touched object, but also voids between the fingers which can only be filled cognitively, from memory, unless the hands are allowed to move. Normal behaviour is for the initial contact to direct further exploratory movement towards points of interest to clear up ambiguities and make a diagnosis.

The eyes, in contrast, assess the three-dimensional world from what is essentially a two-dimensional image. In vision this two-dimensional image is enriched by light and shade, and contains modulations and gradients of colour which are often difficult to analyse and describe, but can nevertheless be interpreted and used by unsophisticated people and by young children.

Contained in this image is perspective information, and sequential information obtained during scanning. Although vision is often described as instantaneous in comparison with touch, this statement is only true in a very loose sense, because slight alterations of image obtained sequentially can yield important information about the shape and orientation of objects in the real world, and about their spatial relationships to one another. Thus, in contrast to touch, our understanding of the three-dimensional world through vision is the result of a translation process from a two-dimensional image, but the voids in the image are not as extensive or as inhibiting as in touch perception.

It is important to stress that blind people using tactile illustrations require a background of rich handling experiences to enable them to understand tactile presentations, and that many teachers and researchers overlook the effect of previous experience in judging the effectiveness of the material they use.

OUTLINE DRAWINGS

People with full vision often see and make use of silhouettes in conditions of poor illumination. Totally blind people never encounter such a flat two-dimensional image. The world encountered by the fingers always has information from the third dimension added to it. Even the suggestion or hint of this third dimension as in, say, a reduced-relief diagram may help the user to interpret the diagram. Accordingly it is found that tactile diagrams which include appropriate textural information, and clear indications of the third dimension, including concave and convex surfaces, will be helpful. In the writer's earlier work on biological tactile diagrams it was found that bold multi-layered relief with convex and concave shapes was needed to convey adequately the rich anatomical information that was sometimes required (Hinton & Ayres 1986; Hinton 1988).

Thus a tactile diagram user may surmise that a structure is shown whole or sectioned according to whether it is depicted with a convex or flat surface. For the same reason concave or sunken channels are often used on a diagram to indicate the presence of a duct or tube, instead of a raised strip or a convex ridge (Hinton, 1988). Although such sunken areas are still uncommon in tactile pictures they are often a more logical and helpful way of dealing with the subject matter, and if of sufficient size, no more difficult to finger-track or interpret.

In tactile form outline drawings can be problematic for the blind user. Pring, a researcher who uses mainly outline drawings in her experimental work, recognises a conflict between "views expressed within the framework of visual perception" and the way the sense of touch operates (Pring, 1987). The writer's classroom experience suggests that with the simple planar diagrams produced on German film (which gives very similar results to the apparatus which Pring used) the ability to identify and interpret a picture depends very much on the form and complexity of the drawing. When this is done successfully without textual or teacher support it is often by the use of relatively superficial features of the drawing, and as Pring discovered, a simple confusion over components of a drawing can lead to early confusion between the stalk of a flower and the handle of a toothbrush (to use Pring's example) (Ibid).

So outline tactile pictures are fraught with difficulty for the blind user. This is not to say that they should not be used, but that teachers and researchers should be aware of their inherent problems and make every possible effort in design and by provision of supporting material to avoid ambiguity and confusion.

TEXTURE AND CONTRAST

Map-makers habitually use standard textures and symbols. In other types of diagram, although standard techniques are used where possible, and it is particularly important that textures for identical structures in a linked series are followed throughout the series, it is not always possible or desirable to adhere to a standard symbol. In such work, it is the diagram CONTEXT which is important, and individual textures are interpreted in relation to what is found around them, (Hinton, 1990; Buultjens, 1988) perhaps with the help of braille or other annotations. Thus, standard textures become less important, but any textures used need to be appropriate and meaningful in the attempt to understand a diagram and its components. In fact, because of the contextual clues which emerge from a diagram a restricted range of textures may not be a problem to the designer.

Just as in vision a preliminary glance over a scene puts closer observations into context, so the first cursory hand scan is important in discovering the meaning of what is on a tactile page. It is therefore possible to manipulate components of a tactile presentation to bring desired features into prominence, thereby helping the reader to isolate those features which are crucial to the understanding of the diagram.

There are three main contrasts which are available to the designer for this purpose. The first is high and low relief, with higher relief tending to be more prominent. The second is rough and smooth texture, and in general rough texture is the more prominent. Both of these two contrasts are part of the stock-in-trade of most tactile diagram designers. The third contrast which is less commonly used is that between concave, flat, and convex shapes. In this case the prominence comes from the novelty of a particular form amongst its surroundings (Hinton, 1988).

At the most basic level it is these contrasts which a designer is able to use to avoid the figure/ground ambiguity which was a source of confusion for Kennedy and Domander's blind subjects in their use of certain tactile line drawings (Kennedy & Domander 1984).

CONGENITAL BLINDNESS

In the past a great deal has been written about the insurmountable difficulties of congenital blindness. Much of this writing has been unnecessarily pessimistic and some of the statements made about the predicament of the congenitally blind are not in fact borne out by carefully investigated facts (Birns, 1986; Cromer, 1973). Controlled experiments do not suggest that congenital blindness imposes any further limits on a blind person's general performance, given an adequate education, than late blindness, although it is admitted that the congenitally-blind person works against a sensory shortfall which needs to be overcome by careful provision. It is also clear that there are individual differences in performance which over-ride the late blind/congenitally blind division. Some of these may be the result of differences in earlier educational experiences (Tobin, 1972).

It was a commonly held belief among some teachers and others, including the less-fortunate congenitally blind people of an earlier generation, that "the congenitally-blind cannot understand tactile diagrams" but careful work and observations under conditions which are fair to the blind person show that this is far from the truth. The present writer has worked with some congenitally blind teenagers and younger children who are highly-proficient in using diagrammatic forms of representation, not only as an aide-memoire after careful schooling, but freely, imaginatively, and with genuine understanding. Many congenitally blind people of an older generation went through a more didactic educational system in which rote-learning was a notable feature. When they complain of difficulties with diagrams, their complaints need to be taken very seriously and met with sympathy and tact, but in the writer's experience rarely denote an insurmountable lack of ability. There is simply a lack of the type of preparatory experience which would lead to success.

MEMORY AND TACTUAL EXPERIENCE

Any perception based on tactual input has two components - a sensory component and a memory component. Even if other modes of sensory input are excluded, the haptic sensations arriving at the central nervous system only partly account for what is perceived, because these sensations are integrated with the subject's memory of previous experience, (most powerfully with previous TACTUAL experience) and are then attended-to, identified, evaluated and responded-to in the light of this experience. It follows that variations in previous experience may be expected to modify the perception. It also follows that any outside influence or supplementary information which may alter the subject's expectations will also have a marked effect on the perception.

In an experiment where blind children from four to six years old attempted to identify familiar objects when the amount of finger contact was artificially restricted to a brief contact by the tip of the index finger and the opposing thumb (Hinton, 1991), the identifications were unanimous, and yet plainly, complete identification of the items given would not be possible from the restricted contact allowed without considerable previous handling experience of the objects. To put it another way, it would be impossible to construct a perception of these objects from the available sensations alone.

Similar results are found with tactile diagrams and pictures and the result will vary according to the richness of the subject's previous experience and the extent to which this is relevant to the picture or can be brought to bear upon the picture. By careful design what is provided on the page may derive the utmost advantage from what is contributed from memory.

In general diagrams there may be a variety of responses to what is on the page and these are often so specific to the subject matter that no useful purpose would be served by quoting individual examples, but to attempt some systematisation of these, consider three possible cases:
(a) Diagram not met before by subject, nor any similar diagram.
(b) Diagram not met before, but similar or related diagram has been used previously.
(c) Diagram or an exact copy met before.

The normal results from these three possible situations appear to be as follows:

(a) The subject will understand the diagram if it bears some similarity to objects from his/her real world and this similarity is sufficiently obvious to the touch. The wider the subject's handling experience, particularly if this has included tactile pictures, the more proficient is he/she likely to be.

(b) Similar results to case (a) with greater chance of success the more obvious the similarities are. Any clues from braille titles, tape or oral instruction will enhance the effect of the diagram.

(c) Recognition can be instantaneous from very slight contact. There is frequently no need for full scanning of the picture. Serial reading of the shapes as in reading lines of braille is not required.

Almost instantaneous identification can result from contact with a tactile picture, but it needs to be emphasised that such a quickness of identification is only possible if the blind person is prepared to risk what Susannah Millar of Oxford University describes as "a trade-off between speed and accuracy". The subject relies on the picture (or object) not possessing bizarre and unpredictable distortions in the spaces between the finger contacts.

This behaviour also accords with general information theory in which *expected* sequencing or juxtapositioning of elements discovered can help to narrow down the number of possibilities to be eliminated, and thus reduce the information-processing load (Attneave, 1959, Chapt.2), as can the possibility of aggregating the information into easily-remembered groups or patterns, which also assists memory (Ibid).

The operation of the mind in this sort of context was summed up in a quotation from Maximus Tyrius, quoted by Ernst Gombrich (1960) the art historian:

"The mind, having received of sense a small beginning of remembrance, runneth on infinitely, remembring all what is to be remembred." Maximus Tyrius, Philosophumena.

When we are presented with a mass of sensory information which at first seems to be formless we try to discover some pattern or rhythm in it; to make some sort of sense out of it.

This is something we try to do from birth and the school of Gestalt Psychology is founded upon this phenomenon. Visual art makes use of this behaviour for successful communication of many creative ideas.

With tactile pictures, as with visual art, the reader's memory and imagination can be stimulated in such a way that they can be encouraged to run ahead, and even perceive things that are not really present at all. In this way tactile communication can be enriched.

THE NOMAD AUDIO-TACTILE DEVICE

Anyone working with tactile illustrations soon realises that the braille annotation which accompanies a diagram is a major problem. Because of the unavoidable space which the braille script takes up it comes to dominate what is on the page, in the mind of the diagram designer if not overtly in the finished product. Much of the braille can be kept off the illustration if key letters are sited on or near the diagram components and further information attached in a separate alphabetic or textural key. If this procedure is carried out carefully by someone who understands the process it can be a useful approach, but wherever the text is divorced from the diagram there is always some disruption to the referencing of one to the other.

In his Nomad Audio-Tactile Device, Parkes (1988) overcomes this problem by providing spoken information in close proximity to the diagram or picture components.

Nomad is a very flexible teaching and learning tool which is specifically designed to be used by totally blind students who can also store their own information for use with the diagram and picture overlays. It is based on a touch-sensitive tablet with voice synthesizer, connected as an add-on to an ordinary desk top computer. Using this device, teacher and student can store information in computer memory which can be re-called by touch through an appropriate tactile diagram overlay placed on top of the tablet.

The Nomad pad is in fact an array of 120 X 80 input switches giving 9600 addressable coordinates which are identifiable by the Nomad circuitry when addressing information recalled from Nomad "files" held on the hard disk of the PC. The resolution of the pressure points on the pad is therefore 5mm, which is less than the size of a human finger. The communication baud rate for Nomad is 4800 Baud for the software versions up to Version 3.1, although the developers recommend a rate of 9600 Baud for Version 4 (which is not yet on general release).

There are only four control buttons on the tablet itself and two of these do most of the work, roughly corresponding to the "enter" key and the "escape" key of a computer. Verbal input is generally by means of the Qwerty keyboard of the attached computer. The tablet functions as a tactile menu array when necessary and can also be primed with the necessary filing information for tactile graphic overlays selected from the catalogue of files already in computer memory.

In our experience many diagrams contain features which are either too complex for the unskilled diagram designer to handle effectively, or require three-dimensional information and for these the microcapsule format does not provide an adequate diagram. Because of this we continue to provide thermoforms as well as microcapsule diagrams for many educational purposes.

Nomad with its direct speech presentation stimulated by the finger which explores the diagram overlay by touch can make the subject matter of a diagram very clear and can even compensate for structural inadequacies in the diagram itself. If to this is added the possibility of harnessing the calculating power of the computer and Nomad's ability to search for a required item the result is a very flexible learning resource. It is also possible to include two additional levels of information which can be recovered during the scanning mode simply by pressing the space bar of the computer keyboard once or twice. So the basic information for the preliminary scan of the diagram can be held on level zero and further layers of information of greater depth or complexity can be added, or a level can be reserved for the student's own responses.

Such a facility permits the use of an overlay which although well-designed and cleansed from all un-necessary clutter still carries information of a complexity which could not be handled in a stand-alone diagram. However much the designer separates out and simplifies material in preliminary teaching diagrams there is still a need to bring large amounts of information together on one page from time to time to describe an overall framework and explain relationships of one part to another. This is important for those with full vision, but it is even more important for a blind student, whose observations are mainly made by touch and can so easily become fragmented in space and in time.

We have used Nomad in teaching in Secondary and Primary schools and with blind university students. One totally-blind ecology student followed a soil science course with the help of a soil map on Nomad without aid. He was provided with a start-up disc for the PC which took him straight into the Nomad environment and from that point he could cope with the spoken Nomad menus.

EARCONS

The development of non-verbal audio-messages (for which the term earcons has been coined) in user-computer interfaces has been stimulated by concern for visual overload, but these signals also potentially offer another means of access to information for the blind user. They are an audio counterpart of the icon. It is a sad fact that while the use of icons in visual interfaces has made computer use easier for the person with full vision this development has made computer access MORE difficult for the visually impaired user.

Blattner et al (1989) describe in some detail the ways in which earcons can be linked in families to denote related operations. They also discuss the relative values and uses of representational and abstract earcons. Earcons can employ many of the features of music in a more direct form. There are thus all the resources of rhythm, pitch, register, timbre and dynamic to make the earcons recognizable and memorable. Memorability is of course a desirable feature if earcons are to have any practical value at the computer interface.

Blattner et al claim the following advantages for their earcon system:
(1) It is systematic and modular and so can be modified and expanded.
(2) Motives can be transformed, combined, or inherited to create families.
(3) Motives can be grouped into families, where earcons with similar meanings have similar sounds while different families can be made to sound disssimilar.
(4) The approach is implementable on most contemporary computer systems.

Simple and compound earcons can have meanings attached to them in the most appropriate way for a given operation. For example, one-note or single-motive earcons are probably best used for the most commonly occuring operations. Compound earcons may be made by *combining* several earcons in succession or by *inheriting* earcons (a term used by the authors for musical factors not occuring in simple succession); the earcons can also be *transformed* to bear a new or modified meaning (the transformation may utilise musical techniques such as inversion, transposition etc.)

The earcons can be made memorable by association as in the use of a volume crescendo for increasing urgency. In fact the Blattner team suggest that in error messages rhythm, pitch and timbre are used to denote the error family, leaving dynamics and register free for modifying the signals for other purposes.

The complexity of the signal is obviously a factor in determining how practical an earcon is in use. Blattner et al (Ibid) use the term "space complexity" for the amount of human memory required to retain an earcon. It is clear that if an earcon is to be of the greatest value it "should convey the necessary information while requiring the user to remember as little as possible, yet the result should not be unpleasant nor fatiguing."

Plainly there is a great deal of scope for the use of earcons as signals at the human/comp[uter interface and they could be beneficial to most users, but especially to the blind user. There is still a great deal to be learned about their efficiency, memorability and how they can be assembled and recognised in combined earcons.

REFRESHABLE DEVICES FOR TACTILE GRAPHICS

There are a number of possible mechanisms being developed at present and these are in various states of progress. So far there is a big gap between the standard of teaching material required if blind students are to do well at school or university, and what has been achieved by these refreshable tactile arrays. However, most of this work is at a very early stage and its potential is high. As was mentioned in discussion of Parkes' Nomad device, this kind of device, particularly with speech output can help to make sense of a tactile display which is less than perfect in the strict tactile sense. It is also vitally important that blind users have effective access to the latest information technology, including that which is displayed in pictorial form.

Although there are a number of research groups working on a variety of designs, most of the devices that have been publicly exhibited have been at the small scale development stage. Up to the Summer of 1992 the author had only seen one such device which approximated to A4 paper size and was therefore capable of carrying an informative graphic. This was the device shown at the Quinquennial Conference of the International Council for the Education of the Visually Handicapped in 1992 by Metec of Stuttgart.

It was based on the same manufacturers moving braille cells, a large number of which had been aggregated into a rectangle and covered with a thin cotton membrane to smooth out the contours of the pins.

This particular device was used to display graph traces, which it did rather indistinctly.

Kruppa's proposed device (Kruppa, 1990) uses an array of low-friction bronze pins of square section with rounded ends where the pins are actually in close contact with each other unlike the last-mentioned device. The drive capsules are separately mounted below and move the pins by means of very fine Bowden cables. Another potentially useful feature of this mechanism is the ability to control each pin at several different heights so that elaborate tactile arrays could be produced.

Kruppa (Ibid) proposes to use this device with video-camera input and then adapt the camera with interchangeable colour filters to allow calculated colour distortion in the expectation that blind users may thereby identify the original colours of images viewed. Kruppa describes his mechanism as a "thesis for the proposed device" and does not record to what extent this has been made into a working prototype.

The mechanism of Shinohara et al.(1991) consists of a temporary tactile display wich generates relief patterns. It appears to be already working on a scale of 16X16 pins on a square matrix. The drive motors are staggered on three levels vertically to save horizontal space and minimise the lost space between the pins. They appear to have reduced this to 1mm. The pins can be raised to a total of 5mm in steps of 0.25mm. So far this device has been used to display simple icons pre-prepared on a PC keyboard and recalled from the memory of the computer.

This research team has done parallel research on object recognition through this type of pin matrix using clay relief models to control the pins, cutting-out the need for computer apparatus. (Saida et al, 1991) Their results, though interesting are at a very early stage at the time of writing.

Minagawa et al (1991) have produced a similar array of pins. Their system for inputting information using the computer keyboard and the output pins together was successfully used by a blind student. They were also able to produce spoken output from their system. They tried out the system with a simple route map.

The mechanism developed by Fricke and Bahring (1991) uses cylinders of electrorheological fluid to control the "up" or "down" state of pre-formed pimples in an elastic membrane over the cylinders. The state of the fluid in each cylinder is controlled by two thin electrodes on the lining of the tube. If both electrodes are connected to a voltage source the cylinder remains in the quiet state, whereas if one is connected to earth the fluid state is changed, the pressure rises and the "pimple" is raised. Unfortunately, as one of these electrodes is connected to the control circuit by a column collection line and the other by a row collection line, control of each cylinder is not fully independent. They can only have their state changed in rectangular areas.

It is important that these and future designers of refreshable tactile displays maintain their dialogue with educational and psychological researchers whose work will continue to direct their developments in effective and appropriate directions.

REFERENCES

Attneave F. (1959), *Applications of Information Theory to Psychology*, New York: Henry Holt

Birns S. L. (1986), Age at Onset of Blindness and Development of Space Concepts: From Topological to Projective Space, *Journal of Visual Impairment and Blindness, 80, (2)*, p.577-582.

Blattner M.M., Sumikawa D.A. & Greenberg R.M. (1989), Earcons and Icons: Their Structure and Common Design Principles, *Human-Computer Interaction, 4*, p.11-44.

Buultjens M. (1988), Computer-based Raised Diagram Designs, in *Proceedings of the Second International Symposium on Maps and Graphics for Visually Handicapped People*, edited by Tatham, A. F., & Dodds, A. G. London: King's College.

Cromer R. F. (1973), Conservation by the Congenitally Blind, *British Journal of Psychology, 64, (2)*, p.241-250.

Fricke J. & Bahring H. (1992), A Graphic Input/Output Tablet for Blind Computer Users, *Proceedings of 3rd International Conference on Computers for Handicapped Persons 7-9th July 1992*, Vienna, p.172-179.

Gombrich E. H. (1960), *Art and Illusion*, Oxford: Phaidon Press.

Hinton R. A. L. (1988), *New Ways with Diagrams: a Handbook for Teachers and Lecturers*, London: RNIB.

Hinton R. A. L. (1990), The Use of Tactile Pictures in Communicating the Work of the Visual Artists to Blind People, *Journal of Visual Impairment and Blindness, 85, (4)*, p.174-175.

Hinton R. A. L. (1991), An Assessment of the Effectiveness of Tactile Presentations as Substitutes for Pictures, *PhD Thesis, Loughborough University of Technology*

Hinton R. & Ayres D. (1986), A Collection of Tactile Diagrams for First Examinations in Biology: Construction and Evaluation, *British Journal of Visual Impairment, IV, (1)*, p.13-16.

Kennedy J. M. & Domander R. (1984), Pictorial Foreground/Background Reversal Reduces tactual recognition by Blind Subjects, *Journal of Visual Impairment and Blindness, 79, (5)*, p.215-216.

Kruppa L. (1990), Graphical Display for Tactile Perception, *Journal of Microcomputer Applications, 13*, p.165-176.

Millar S. (1975), Visual Experience or Translation Rules? Drawing the Human Figure by Blind and Sighted Children, *Perception, 4*, p.363-373.

Minagawa H., Ohnishi N. & Sugie N., (1992), A Vision Substitution System for Reading and Writing Diagrams Using Tactile and Auditory Senses, in *Proceedings of 3rd International Conference on Computers for Handicapped Persons*, 7-9th July 1992, Vienna, p.353-362.

Parkes D. (1988), Nomad: an Audio-tactile tool for the acquisition, use and management of spatially distributed information by visually impaired people, in *Proceedings of the Second International Symposium on Maps and Graphics for Visually Handicapped People*, ed. Tatham, A. F. & Dodds, A.G. London: King's College.

Pring L. (1987), Picture Processing by the Blind, *British Journal of Educ. Psychology*, 57, p.38-44.

Saida S., Shinohara M., Shimizu Y., Esaka Y. & Shimura H. (1992), Development of a 3-D Tactile Display for the Blind: Preferable Presentation, in *Proceedings of 3rd International Conference on Computers for Handicapped Persons*, 7-9th July 1992, Vienna, p;431-437.

Shinohara M., Saida S., Shimuzu Y., Mochizuku A. & Sorimachi M. (1992), Development of a 3-D Tactile Display for the Blind: System Design, in *Proceedings of 3rd International Conference on Computers for Handicapped Persons*, 7-9th July 1992, Vienna, p.422-430.

Tobin M. (1972), Conservation of Substance in the Blind, *British Journal of Educ. Psychology*, 42, (2), p.192-197.

Résumé

L'information qu'il est possible d'obtenir d'une image visuelle est fort différente de celle que donne une image tactile. Cet article souligne les limitations et les ambiguïtés inhérentes à la réalisation de dessins en relief. Il explique dans quelle mesure l'utilisation de textures et de contrastes peut être mise à profit pour minimiser ce problème. Il insiste sur l'importance de la mémoire dans la perception par le toucher. Les besoins des jeunes aveugles de naissance en matière de documents pour l'enseignement sont particulièrement discutés.

Le système Nomad, fondé sur un principe audio-tactile, est présenté. D'autres recherches techniques visant à produire des systèmes permettant la restitution de formes en relief sont évoquées. Bien que leur utilisation à des fins pédagogiques apparaisse encore limitée, leur potentiel pour l'avenir est souligné.

Mathematical representations: graphs, curves and formulas

Alistair D.N. Edwards and Robert D. Stevens

Department of Computer Science, University of York, York YO1 5DD, United Kingdom

ABSTRACT

Mathematics is communicated in visual forms, such as algebra and diagrams. This means that blind people are greatly disadvantaged with respect to education and employment in mathematics, science and technology. A number of ideas are presented regarding the representation of mathematics in non-visual formats. In particular, the *Mathtalk* software for the presentation of algebra in synthetic speech, is described, as is *Soundgraph* a program which presents the graphs of mathematical functions in speech and non-speech sounds.

INTRODUCTION

Mathematics is the foundation of most science and technology. There is a language in which mathematics is communicated and that language is inherently visual. Hence a visual disability can be a bar to the study and use of mathematics, and this is a very serious exclusion since it also affects access to science and technology. This paper sets out to demonstrate that there are alternative, non-visual means of communicating mathematics, based on the use of interactive computers and multiple, non-visual communication modes. It is also suggested, however, that significant further research will be required before the full potential of these forms of communication will be realized.

Speech is the richest form of non-visual communication, but it has limitations with respect to the presentation of mathematical information. One significant limitation is that speech (as with all sounds) is *transient*; it is impossible to review an utterance. (The nearest one can get to doing that is to review an internal representation of the utterance, a memory of it – which may be incomplete). Also the *words* of a language convey limited amounts of information. For most purposes efficient communication is achieved only by additional, non-verbal channels. So in spoken language, the *prosody* conveys extra meaning: whether a question is implied, or the speaker wishes to convey irony, for instance.

Such are the limitations of speech, but written natural language is also insufficiently powerful to express mathematical ideas; it is too verbose. Therefore a written language which is much more compact for expressing mathematical concepts has evolved, and that language is known as algebra. Algebra is very powerful because it makes use of a very rich set of symbols and (two-dimensional) spatial relationships between them. It is fundamentally a written language because those spatial relationships cannot easily be expressed in speech which is essentially one-dimensional[1]. Thus, whenever two mathematicians meet, there is usually a piece of paper or a blackboard not far away. Only with that visual medium can they communicate unambiguously.

Mathematics is a compulsory subject in schools. Many people find its study hard and undertake it for as short a time as possible. To such people, exclusion from mathematics is seen not as a handicap, but probably a positive escape. However, for anyone who wishes to pursue studies and a career in *any* technological or scientific field, continued access to mathematics is essential. In other words, anyone who cannot read and write mathematics for any reason is excluded from a high proportion of career alternatives. Throughout this paper, when reference is made to mathematicians, the reader should bear in mind that the person referred to might well not be a mathematician as such, but an engineer, physicist, chemist, teacher *etc*. A particular example is that the advent of accessible computers has created a population of blind people with an interest in computers, but for most of them the academic study of Computer Science is precluded partly because of their lack of mathematics qualifications.

One of the beauties of mathematical languages is that they are international. Although mathematicians annotate any discussions in their native language, the formula

$$x = \frac{-b \pm \sqrt{(b^2 - 4ac)}}{2a} \qquad [1]$$

should be as meaningful to any French-speaking mathematician as to an English-speaker. So, while it may be suggested that the number of blind mathematicians is a small, and hence that the payoff of this area of research will be small, there is a counter-argument that world-wide that number is large and that the smallest progress in the field will be of broadest significance. This multi-lingual character makes this an almost ideal area for research within the European Community.

Ironically 'doing' mathematics is essentially an intellectual activity, carried out 'in the head'. It is only when one wants to communicate a mathematical idea that one hits the barrier of its visual nature. (Though it is also important to bear in mind that most mathematicians need to communicate not only with others, but also with themselves. In other words, writing down intermediate results can be very important. This is discussed further below). Thus, a person may be intellectually perfectly well equipped to understand and perform mathematics, but simply lack the means of communicating it.

---

[1] One should be wary of making this assertion too glibly. As will be argued later, sounds can be used which have many more than one dimension and a major research interest is in what other dimensions exist and how best to exploit them.

Although the above discussion has related mainly to algebra, this is not the only (visual) mathematical language. A large number of diagrammatical representations exist. They all have their particular features and strengths, but there is no reason why they should not be transformed to other, non-visual forms.

We have also concentrated so far on auditory presentation, which is the main focus of our work at York. However, we do recognize that either the tactile or auditory sense may be used. It is also possible to exploit different *modalities* of communication on any channel. For instance, greater use can be made of the hearing channel if both verbal and non-verbal modalities are used. Each modality has its strengths and weaknesses. In general one wants to exploit the strengths, and often the best way of doing this is to make as many modalities available as possible – and allow the user to choose.

Braille is the traditional substitute for printed text for blind people, and mathematical braille codes have been developed. There are a number of features of braille which make it superior to auditory communication. Notably braille is *persistent*; the reader has the possibility of passing backwards and forwards through the text. However, braille also has some limitations. Currently the greatest short-coming of mathematical braille is the lack of standardization of braille codes, but work is proceeding on this topic (Wesley and Wallace, 1992).

This paper is concerned with the development of auditory representations of mathematics, but – as suggested above – ultimately the ideal mathematics interface for blind users will have as many modalities of communication as possible. Currently the greatest obstacle to the exploitation of the variety of communications channels and modalities is our lack of understanding of how to use them. As Alty (1991) pointed out, we know very little about how to use any of the new modalities in isolation, far less how best to use them in multi-modal combinations.

SOUNDS AND ACCESS TO COMPLEX INFORMATION

The rate of transmission of information – in both directions – between the computer and the user is often referred to as the *bandwidth*. Human visual bandwidth is relatively large. This means that the designers of visual interfaces can cram a lot of information on a computer screen all (or most) of which is constantly visible to the user. This highly parallel presentation of information is not overwhelming because the user can rapidly switch attention to the current point of interest and ignore or filter out any extraneous information. Problems occur when the bandwidth is not sufficient for a particular application.

The basic problem of adapting any visual interface for blind people is that none of the other senses has as broad bandwidth as vision. It has been suggested above that a great deal more work will have to be done before we start to make anything like full use of the potential bandwidth of non-speech sounds. Yet, even when something like that full bandwidth has been realized, it will still not match that available in vision. There are two possible approaches to this problem. One is to reduce the amount of information presented, to filter it through the narrow bandwidth channel. The other is to attempt to broaden the total bandwidth by making use of other senses in combination with hearing. The hope is that the whole will be greater than the sum of the parts, that in combining media and modes of presentation, new channels of communication will be discovered.

There are three projects under way at York in this field, and the hope is to expand them into a large-scale research project. One is looking at the presentation of mathematics in synthetic speech and the second is concerned with translating simple diagrams (line graphs) into sounds. The third project is concerned with combining non-visual media and modes.

PRESENTATION OF ALGEBRA IN SPEECH

Mathematicians have to use algebra to communicate because they have to be able to convey a great deal of information and it must be precise. Whereas in conversational speaking or writing the odd word mis-heard does not generally affect the understanding, one symbol missed in algebra can completely alter the meaning of the expression. Written algebra relies on the reader's ability to scan, move backwards and forwards and to focus on the relevant terms, in other words it relies on all the properties of vision which make it so powerful. In translating algebra into a non-visual form it is desirable to substitute for as many of these properties as possible. It is *not* sufficient to simply send a stream of text to a speech synthesizer and have it spoken as one long utterance. There must be the ability to *control* the way the expression is scanned and spoken.

The objective of this project is to see how to exploit a variety of communication modes to present algebra in a meaningful manner. This involves not only using several auditory modalities, but also designing the interaction such that the person is aware of the structure of the expressions being viewed.

In written algebra the printed form helps the reader in several ways. The two-dimensional nature of algebra notation delimits syntactic groups by their spatial location. Exponents and fractions are good examples of this. These are visually obtrusive parsing markers. Additionally, the spacing of the symbols on the page aids parsing in a more implicit way. The order of precedence of algebraic operators can be correlated with the spatial arrangement. This 'visual syntax' (Kirshner, 1989) helps a significant number of readers to successfully parse an expression. A reader can review an expression and quickly focus attention on any part. The ability to perceive the expression as a whole has implications for the manipulation of an expression. A user's perception of an expression's structure will guide his or her strategy in solving the current problem. (Lewis, 1981).

A reader of print is able to control the information flow, through the ability to browse an expression. This facility needs to be offered to the person who 'reads' an expression with speech. Given the amount of information available, there is a need to *filter* it for comprehension. Vision is very well adapted to such filtering tasks, because attention can be focused on the salient parts. To present the same information in an auditory form, it is necessary for the computer to perform the filtering task.

However, this filtering must not be prescriptive; the reader must maintain control over which parts of the information are revealed at any time, and must never be excluded access to any part.

There are two problems to be addressed. One is to devise facilities which will give the user access to all the information available in a visual system and the second problem is, having identified the forms in which to present the information, to enable the user to control that access. In this section we describe progress on solving the former problem in the context of the presentation of algebra, but as yet there is less to be said about the latter. As explained above, the amount of information available is very large. Having retained it all in an auditory form, the interface through which it will be controlled is necessarily complex.

Whereas reading is an active process, listening is a passive one. Reading aloud is relatively slow, and a listener is liable to lose concentration. However, in a one-to-one situation, a listener may be able to take a more active part in the reading process. A skilled reader, using meaningful symbol names and unambiguous speech, can interpret the structure of an expression to deliver it in a controlled and comprehensible manner. In such cases a listener can interact and direct the reader in the same process.

It should be possible to replace the human reader with an interactive computer system. Such a system must be able to speak an expression, via a voice synthesizer, in a consistent and unambiguous way. The listener becomes a reader and should be able to use an overview of an expression's structure to guide his or her interaction. This interaction must enable the user to comprehend the macro-structure and detail of an expression and the relationship between its structural components, much as the reader of print is able.

The first decision in speaking algebra notation is what type of information to give the reader. The written form gives the reader a literal meaning of an expression. The interpretation of that expression to something of more focused mathematical meaning relies on the user's knowledge. For instance, the expression

$$E = mc^2$$

can be interpreted at a number of different levels. It may simply be judged as a set of relationships between items, a quantity labelled E is equal to the product of two other quantities, m and c^2. A more sophisticated mathematician would be able to make other inferences about the properties implied by the equation (such as what a plot of E versus m would look like). However, a physicist would probably recognize a much more important interpretation: that mass and energy are equivalent.

The point here is that it is the *literal* meaning of an expression that should be presented, not any interpretation. However, the expression should be presented in such a way that the reader can apply his or her knowledge to the information and make an interpretation. For instance, it is a relatively simple matter to produce a computer program which will solve a set of simultaneous equations, but that is not what is required. Rather the user needs the tools by which he or she can solve them.

Chang (1983) has devised a set of guidelines for the reading of mathematics such that ambiguity is eliminated. Firstly he offers a set of standard names for symbols, but a more significant aspect of the system is its facilities for delimiting certain groups of symbols within an expression by the use of key-words and phrases. These groups of symbols are those delimited, in print, by spatial location or visually obtrusive markers, such as fractions and parentheses.

For example, parentheses are replaced with the words 'the quantity' and 'end quantity'. Similarly the phrases: 'the fraction', 'the numerator', 'the denominator' and 'end fraction', are used to delimit the scope of a fraction-line. Such phrases replace parsing markers such as parenthesis (which is difficult to say) and spatial cues such as superscripts and vertical juxtaposition in fractions. In this way a listener is given the structure in an unambiguous fashion, by explicitly starting and ending certain syntactic structures. Using Chang's method, equation [1] would be read as:

> *X equals the fraction, numerator negative b plus or minus the square root of the quantity b squared minus 4 a c, denominator 2 a.*

The idea of simple and complex notation can be introduced to explain the use of these delimiting phrases. Complexity arises when grouping symbols are needed to prevent syntactic ambiguity, when an expression is written in a linear form. For example, $x^{(n+1)}$. Here the parentheses explicitly place both terms following the x into the superscript and the phrase 'end power' is needed in the spoken form. In contrast to this complex example, a single term in the superscript requires no explicit termination. Similarly, a simple fraction, such as $\frac{x}{y}$ can be spoken as 'x over y', but complex fraction, $\frac{x+y}{x-y}$ needs to have the verbal tags inserted (i.e. the fraction, numerator x plus y, denominator x - y).

Such guidelines for the speaking of algebra only solve one aspect of the problem, and may exacerbate another. The addition of many verbal tags could increase the, already large, cognitive load on a listener, further preventing a proper reading of the expression. This point reinforces the need for the listener to be able to control the information flow.

Another important feature of spoken algebra must be introduced at this point. The intonation pattern or prosody of a person's voice contains important information above the purely lexical content. Perceived pauses and the pitch change within speech divide the utterance into 'units of information, new and given' (Halliday 1970) and focus attention on certain items within those units. Prosody can give structure to an utterance, indicating major syntactic boundaries. A preliminary investigation has revealed some relatively simple rules for the prosody of algebra. Pauses are inserted at major syntactic boundaries, speed and pitch change also emphasize a change in structure. The use of these cues in spoken algebra could aid the process known as chunking. Additionally, some of the verbal tags could be replaced with prosodic cues. Another significant prosodic feature seems to be a sharp decrease in the pitch contour at the end of an expression. This feature could be useful to indicate the end of an expression.

The addition of prosody to speech amounts to adding another, non-verbal modality to the speech communication channel. The extent to which it will be useful depends to a great extent on how authentically it can be produced by a speech synthesizer. Experiments are proceeding attempting to implement the prosody rules on a variety of synthesizers.

As the complexity of an expression can indicate where to place verbal cues within an expression, it can also guide the control of information flow. Besides the full uttering of an expression, three modes of browsing an expression have been devised. These are *unconstrained*, *unfolding* and *staged release* browsing.

A full utterance is adequate when the amount of information is small enough to be retained and integrated, that is to say that it is 'simple'. When the expression becomes too complex, through length or syntactic construction, other views need to be presented. Unconstrained browsing allows movement through an expression, character to character, term to term, into and out of complex items, etc. The reader can ask for a range of views to be spoken. These include, character term, superscript, level, complex structure etc. This browsing style allows a detailed examination of an expression. If a reader finds a spoken expression too long to remember, a staged release strategy may be used. Each term is spoken in turn upon request. Staged release browsing would not be appropriate for equation [1] since it is too complex. It might be used (for instance) for a quadratic of the form

$$ax^2 + bx + c$$

since each of the terms is simple. Staged release would allow the user to hear each of those terms one at a time.

This control enables the expression to be broken into manageable units, that readers can retain and integrate at their own pace. The last browsing type is an unfolding strategy. In this method a series of views, ever more complex, are given to the reader. In each view simple syntax is spoken, until a complex structure is found. This complex item is referred to by its type, 'quantity' or 'fraction'. At the next signal from the reader the complex item is spoken as before. At the end of the complex structure, speaking commences again, at the previous level, upon a signal from the reader. Using unfolding browsing, equation [1] might be read as follows (where a gap indicates that the user must signal that he or she is ready for the next component).

X equals a fraction;

numerator negative b plus or minus the square root of a quantity;

b squared minus 4 a c;

denominator 2 a.

The choice between a full utterance, unconstrained browsing, unfolding or a staged release is the choice of how to filter the information flow. The different browsing strategies reflect the structural nature of an expression and the presentation type reinforces that structure for the user. Naturally, the user can switch between browsing strategies at any time. The control also enables the reader to read at his or her own pace.

To make a sensible choice between browsing strategies a reader has to have some idea of the overall structure, complexity or macro-syntax of an expression. This is one aspect of the very information the reader is attempting to acquire. The verbal reader needs a 'glance at' or summary of the essential features of an expression in order to make that choice. The ability of prosody to impart the syntactic structure of an expression indicates a possibility to impart an overview to a listener. In essence, by giving the listener the prosodic structure of a skilled speaker's reading, the algebraic structure can be given. Just as spatial location on the page aids the parsing of an expression, so can the pattern of pauses, pitch and speed change within the speaking of an expression. This idea of 'prosody without the speech' can be achieved using non-speech audio.

These abstract representations of prosodic structure are called *algebra earcons*, based upon earcons, as described in Brewster, Wright and Edwards (1993), Brewster (1991) and Blattner, Sumikawa and Greenberg (1989). This represents the use of another auditory modality.

An interactive computer implementation of this reading method is currently being developed. The *Mathtalk* program can present the core of algebra notation (input in the *Tex*, text-processing format, Knuth, 1987), to an arbitrary complexity. The speech style, based on that of Chang, is consistent and unambiguous. The unconstrained, unfolding and staged-release browsing strategies have also been implemented. The algebra prosody and algebra earcons in the process of being implemented.

The system as a whole, should enable a listener, to read an expression more actively. Selection of a browsing strategy, based on the complexity of an expression, presents a series of expression views, best suited to convey the syntax of the expression. The prosody of algebra plays two roles in the system.

Once algebra has been transformed into an auditory format, as described, there will remain the problem of providing the user with an interface through which to control access to the information. All the information of the visual format is retained. In fact there is redundancy in that the same components of an expression can be viewed in different ways, using the alternative browsing strategies. Given that amount of information, the interface to it is necessarily going to be complex. A command language has been developed to enable the user to control the presentation of information. Two words make one command, the first is an *action* and the second word a *target*. The initial letters of these command words are mapped mnemonically onto the keyboard. Action words include 'next', 'previous', 'current', 'start' and 'quit'. These actions work upon targets such as 'character', 'term', 'level', 'sub-expression' and 'expression'. This command language is universal within the system. For example, in the main menu, 'next+expression' moves to the next expression in the list. The action 'start' with the target 'unfolding', will put the user into the browsing mode. The command 'quit+expression' removes a user from a browsing mode.

In developing this system, other, wider questions of computer interaction by visually disabled users will have to be tackled. These include command selection, feedback, navigation and orientation.

Presentation of information about the system, by the system is difficult. To select a suitable command from a menu is necessarily slow in speech, when only one item is visible at a time. The reading process needs to be quick and the command process (issue and feedback) needs to be transparent as possible. A principle followed in this design is to not let issuing commands interfere with the presentation of the algebra. A careful design of the presentation should allow the spoken algebra to provide appropriate feedback for the user. For example, movement right would be associated with a relative fall in pitch, as is the case with a human speaker.

Non-speech audio also has a role to play in indicating start and end of levels and movement between levels. Non-speech audio feedback for errors, by earcons, would decrease the need for disruptive speech messages.

The transient nature of speech means that review of preceding information is difficult. A consequence of this may be a lack of orientation, both within the system and a browsed expression. Suitable context-giving functions will be developed for the system. A combination of algebraic prosody, the browsing functions themselves and non-speech audio should be able to relieve problems of orientation and navigation. By providing this ability in an unobtrusive manner should solve problems and enhance the 'reading' process.

SOUNDGRAPHS

Another visual format for the presentation of mathematical information is the *line graph*. A diagram, such as that in Fig. 1, conveys a great deal of information. As with algebra part of the power of such displays is due to the fact that the user can select the portion of the information contained within it which is pertinent to their current requirements. For instance, in order to answer certain queries, it may be the overall shape of the curve which is of interest, whereas in another context, it may be the point at which the curve crosses the x-axis which is important.

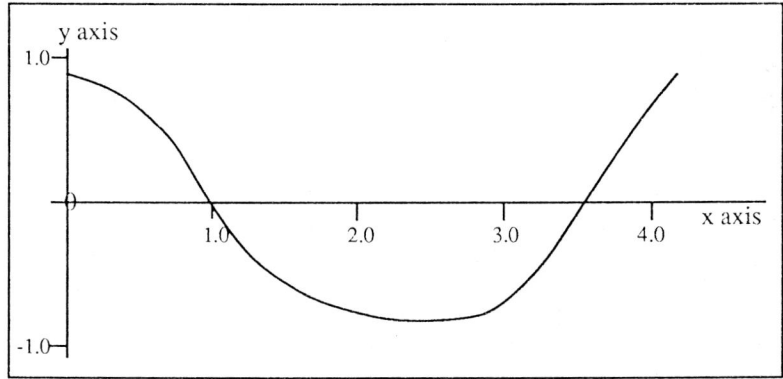

Fig. 1. *A typical line graph. This comprises a lot of information, but a sighted person is able to cope with all that information by focussing in on whichever aspect of it is pertinent to his or her current needs.*

Sound graphs (Mansur, Blattner and Joy, 1985) are an attempt to provide access to such graphical information through the use of non-speech sounds. The idea has been implemented as a software package at York (Pitt and Edwards, 1992). The basic idea of a sound graph is that the y value of the curve should be represented by the pitch of a tone, the x-axis being essentially represented by time.

Soundgraph is multi-modal in that it combines speech and non-speech sounds. It also has a visual display. This was included in order to make the software usable by partially sighted (and indeed normally sighted) people. It turns out that this combination may be significant. Partially sighted people need aids which enable them to make full use of their residual vision.

Hence, most of them prefer not to use non-visual interfaces (such as those which are purely speech-based). In this case, however, they can use a visual interface (possibly with the assistance of a screen enlarger) but they do also receive the auditory feedback which seems to be a helpful augmentation.

Graphs can be played to a listener, giving an indication of their shape, but they can also be examined interactively, so that the user can locate points of interest, such as turning points. The user effectively moves a cursor backwards and forwards along the curve. At any time the note sounded corresponds to the height of the curve at that point. It is possible to enlarge the area around the cursor, to make more accurate location possible and the coordinates of any point on the curve can be obtained in speech. Speech (through a standard screen reader) is also used as the basis of the interaction, to make the package accessible to blind users.

An important feature of Soundgraph is that it not only allows users to view graphs, but also to create them. There are several methods through which this can be done. One is that they may be 'drawn' by the user. Using the same form of pitch and speech feedback as in the interactive display mode, the user can place the cursor at a chosen point in the space and place a point there to be included on the curve. Alternatively should the user want to plot a curve for which they know the function the graph can be created by entering that formula (in a programming-language-like format). Some simple common functions are built in and the user can construct a graph of any of them by providing a few parameters (range of x values, coefficients *etc*). Finally it is possible to import data from other packages (such as spread sheets) in the form of simple text files containing pairs of coordinates.

The Soundgraph software was tested during development, with the assistance of the Royal National Institute for the Blind Vocational Training College and the Royal National for the Blind. A formal evaluation of the finished product is now planned. It was designed to be distributed to schools and colleges and to be accessible on as wide a range of computers as possible[2]. It was therefore implemented on a PC computer, using no special graphics or add-on sound cards. That means that the visual display and sound output are crude. It is planned to produce an enhanced option which will make use of a sound card. See the section on Further Work.

COGNITIVE REPRESENTATIONS AND INTEGRATION OF MEDIA

This project is as yet in its early stages. The plan is to approach the problem of the narrow bandwidth of the non-visual channels by combining them. The hope is that presenting information in parallel in a complementary fashion on more than one channel will increase the bandwidth available. The obstacle to doing that at present is that little is known about what is a 'complementary fashion'. To that end, therefore preliminary work is being carried out to find a model for the cognitive representation that blind users have of interfaces.

---

[2]. Soundgraph can be obtained for a cost of £5 from: Research Centre for the Education of the Visually Handicapped, School of Education, PO Box 363, Birmingham, England B15 2TT

FURTHER WORK

There is much scope for further work in this field. There are many more forms of representation of mathematics than have been mentioned above. Also, apart from Soundgraph's capability to create graphs, the above discussion has been mainly about the *reading* of mathematics, in one form or another. A much more important requirement is for facilities by which the blind mathematician can *manipulate* mathematical objects. It is a sobering thought that what we need to emulate is the simple pad and paper used by sighted mathematicians, yet only the best of minds can pursue a proof without writing down intermediate steps to aid memory and allow inspection.

There is also a need for much greater understanding of the use of non-speech sounds. Bly has demonstrated that complex, multi-dimensional information can be encoded and recognized in sounds. Recent technological developments have also made it possible to generate sounds in three-dimensional space (Wenzel, 1992) which opens many new possibilities. For instance, while manipulating an algebraic formula, the user might be 'immersed' in it, with terms heard to the left and right and above and below, reflecting the printed spatial layout.

More specifically, there is a lot more work to be done on Soundgraph. Whereas the current version was designed to be compatible with the most basic hardware, the addition of a sound card would allow the possibility of experimenting with further use of non-speech sounds. For instance, it has been suggested that a curve could be represented by a varying-pitch sounds, as described above, but that that sound could be augmented by another note, representing the first derivative of the curve. This richer sound would contain more information and might make it easier to locate turning points, for example. Other suggested enhancements include the ability to display two curve simultaneously – or at least to be able to switch quickly between them.

CONCLUSIONS

The advent of computers has opened new possibilities for communication of information through new media and modes. Specifically, it means that there are now alternatives to the traditional printed representation of mathematics and hence improved opportunities for giving blind people access to mathematical material. The work presented in this paper represents early developments in this field and there is still a great deal of work to be done before the full potential will be realized, making maximum use of non-visual communication to communicate the complex information required to perform mathematics. However, the potential benefits are considerable, opening new opportunities in mathematics, science and technology to blind (and partially sighted) people in different countries.

REFERENCES

Alty J. L. (1991), Multimedia – what is it and how do we exploit it? In *People and Computers VI: Proceedings of the HCI'91 Conference*, edited by D. Diaper and N. Hammond, Cambridge University Press, p.31-46.

Blattner M. M., Sumikawa D. A. & Greenberg R. M. (1989), Earcons and icons: Their structure and common design principles, *Human-computer Interaction*, 4 (1), p.11-44.

Bly S. (1982), *Sound and computer information presentation*, PhD Thesis, University of California, Davis, California, USA.

Brewster S. A. (1991), *Providing a model for the use of sound in user interfaces*, University of York, Department of Computer Science, Technical Report YCS169.

Brewster S. A., Wright P. C. & Edwards A. D. N. (1993) An evaluation of earcons for use in auditory human-computer interfaces, *Proceedings of InterChi'93*, (in press).

Buxton (1989), Introduction to the special issue on non-speech audio, *Human-Computer Interaction*, 4(1)p.1-9.

Chang L. A. (1983), *Handbook for spoken mathematics (Larry's Speakeasy)*, Technical Report, Lawrence Livermore Laboratory.

Halliday M. K. (1970), *A course in spoken English: intonation*, Oxford University Press.

Kirshner D. (1989), The Visual Syntax of Algebra, *Journal for Research into Mathematics Education*, 20 (3), p.274-287.

Knuth D. E. (1987), *The Texbook*, Addison-Wesley, Reading, Massachusetts.

Lewis C. (1981), Skill in Algebra Cognitive (in) Anderson, J. R (ed.) *Skills and their Acquisition*, Lawrence Earlbaum Associates, New Jersey.

Mansu D. L., Blattner M. M. & Joy, K. I., (1985), Sound-Graphs: a numerical data analysis method for the blind, *Journal of Medical Systems*, 9, p.163-174.

Pitt I. J. & Edwards A. D. N. (1992), *Final Report on the Nuffield Project, Making Line Graphs Accessible to Blind Students*, Unpublished report, Department of Computer Science, University of York.

Smith S., Grinstein G. G. & Bergeron R. D (1990), Stereophonic and surface sound generation for exploratory data analysis, *Proceedings of CHI'90*, Seattle, Washington, p.125-132.

Wenzel, E M, (1992) Three-dimensional virtual acoustic displays. In *Multimedia Interface Design*, edited by M. M. Blattner and R. B. Dannenberg, Addison-Wesley, New York, p.257-288.

Wesley T. & Wallace J. (1992), The application of information technology to the access of mathematical information for the blind, in Zagler, W. (editor) *Proceedings of the Third International Conference on Computers for Handicapped Persons*, Vienna, p.562–569.

Résumé

La modalité visuelle joue un rôle très important pour la communication en mathématiques. Les personnes aveugles sont donc grandement désavantagées dans les domaines scientifiques et technologiques, qu'il s'agisse de suivre une formation ou d'exercer un emploi. Cet article présente un certain nombre des idées qui peuvent être mises à profit pour représenter de manière non visuelle des éléments mathématiques tels que formules algébriques, courbes ou diagrammes. Le logiciel MathTalk, destiné à présenter des formules algébriques grâce à un synthétiseur de parole est décrit, ainsi que SoundGraph permettant de traduire une courbe de manière auditive, sous une forme à la fois verbale et non-verbale.

Methods of text presentation

Christian Fluhr

INSTN/MIST/SBDS/GITD, CE-Saclay, 91191 Gif/Yvette Cedex, France

ABSTRACT

Texts are now being increasingly used in a computer readable form, so new methods need to be developed to replace the human method of browsing through a text that can only be used in the paper form. This paper describes new attitudes and tools for information retrieval. Such tools use character strings and information about text structure. They thus make it possible to access relevant information. Standards for the coding of structured texts are presented. Then, different types of text manipulation are reviewed and tools which enable people to perform these manipulations are introduced. Both the need for personalisation and the adaptation of interfaces for the blind are also discussed.

INTRODUCTION

This paper describes new attitudes and tools for text manipulation and information retrieval. Texts are now being increasingly used in a computer readable form, so new methods need to be developed to replace the human method of browsing through a text that can only be used in the paper form.

FROM DOCUMENT ARCHIVING TO INFORMATION RETRIEVAL

With the arrival on the market of WORMs (Wright Once Read Many), many computer companies have proposed to archive paper documents on this kind of optical disk. Their large capacity (0.5 to 4 Gigabytes) and the fact that they are removable (a juke box can be used) means that they are suitable for very large files like bitmap images of paper documents. The large volume means that it is necessary to compress this image coding by using compression algorithms.

This kind of product provides a solution to the problem of space necessary for information storage, but not for the problem of easy information retrieval. Of course, most of these systems include a brief description of each document (document references, name, a restricted number of key words, etc...). This kind of description can only be useful if users already know what document they are looking for. We can say that it is a *document retrieval* system.

This may be sufficient for dead archives but it does not suffice for documents containing useful information. In this case, *information retrieval* systems that can precisely locate information inside the documents are needed.

Automatic processing of the text is indispensable because a very precise and deep description of the document content using manual indexing is very expensive.

Unfortunately, the image storage of documents is not suitable for content analysis, so the document must be stored in a form that preserves the content of character strings, information about the structure (title, paragraphs, figures, etc...) and the possibility of reproducing the paper form (if it exists). Character strings are indispensable for automatic indexing which is the only way to locate information precisely. Knowledge about the structure helps automatic indexing and is indispensable for the automatic creation of hypertext links (cross references, access to figures, access from table of contents to parts of the text). Of course, image storage cannot be used in the case of blind readers. Only character strings can be easily converted into speech synthesis or transitory braille. The storage of documents in a character form preserving the structure and the possibility of reproducing the paper document has the advantage of saving storage space because information is more compressed that image storage, even when using a very efficient compression algorithm.

The inconvenience lies in the difficulty of storing old documents when a computer readable form is not available. In this case, OCR (Optical Character Recognition) systems must be used to convert images into character strings. The results can then be processed to detect information about the structure and detect cross-references.

The best solution is to access the document directly by using the tool which produced it (word processor). Because of the diversity of tools and coding, a standard should be used to authorise mixing of documents in a safe retrieval system and to allow the exchange of documents. There are two candidates: SGML and ODA (Danish Standards Association, 1991).

STANDARDS FOR REPRESENTING AND EXCHANGING TEXTS

Before giving information about SGML and ODA, the differences between logical structure and physical structure must be explained.

The *logical structure* is the organisation of the document according to semantic content. It is the author's point of view.

In this structure the document is composed for example of a title, the authors'names and address, a summary and introduction, a list of chapters, each of them divided into subchapters, there are also figures liked to the text, cross references to other parts of the documents or to other documents (references), and also some parts of the text are highlighted because the author considers that they are important words for the understanding of the text.

The *physical structure* gives the document a particular physical aspect. It is the typographer's point of view. A document is composed of pages, the first has the title in a big bold font, the author's name in a different font, the summary in italics, the pages have a height and width, the fonts are different for chapter titles and chapter content, words to be highlighted are in bold characters, pages have two columns, there is a table of contents giving access to each chapter or subchapter, there is an index, etc...As you can see, the physical structure may depend on the logical structure, on the dimension of support (height and width), on the nature of support (paper, screen, speech synthesis), on aesthetic considerations and typographic rules etc...Where as it is now possible for the physical structure to be in the form of an A4 sheet on a computer screen. This method of presentation is not the most suitable since access based on the logical structure could benefit from the increasing power of new software techniques. The logical form is needed both to improve screen reading, and to reproduce the paper document in its original form. In this case, a coding of the particular physical form, or the formatting orders to convert the logical form into the physical one, is necessary.

Two standards are available for representing structured documents. The first is SGML (Standard Generalised Markup Language) which is particularly used and promoted in the world of publishing. It is also used in technical documentation and is part of CALS, a set of standards that must be used by companies working for the US Defense Department.

The other standard is ODA, formerly Office Document Architecture, which is now Open Document Architecture. This standard is mainly promoted by people from the field of Office Automation.

SGML can only describe a logical structure. It is a Markup language because all the parts of documents are delimited by a beginning and ending sequence of characters called markups.

ex: <TI> Text presentation methods </TI>

where <TI> gives the beginning of the Title and </TI> gives the end. Ending markups are often dropped if the situation is unambiguous.

This language is said to be "generalised" because the markups and the structure are not defined for each kind of text, but at the beginning of the SGML file in the form of a grammar called a DTD (Document Type Definition). SGML only provides information about the logical structure, so the transformation to be made must be expressed in order to obtain a particular physical form. A new standard covering this problem is under discussion but has not yet been adopted.

ODA codes both the logical and physical structure. There are no markups in the text as the description of the structure and the text content are separate.

There are currently more tools available for SGML than for ODA, and there are more users. For SGML, word processors, information retrieval systems and structure checkers are available from various companies. ODA has been mainly promoted by big European Computer manufacturers for their strategy in Office Automation.

Example of an SGML DTD for notes

```
<!ELEMENT NOTE --(DATE,AUTHOR+,ADDRESSEE+,CONTENT)>
<!ELEMENT DATE--#PCDATA>
<!ELEMENT (AUTHOR|ADDRESSEE)--(FSTNAME,LSTNAME)>
<!ELEMENT CONTENT--(P+)>
<!ELEMENT (FSTNAME|LSTNAME)--#PCDATA>
```

N.B.: The "+" says that there can be more than one element, for example there can be more than one author or addressee.

Example of a document using the preceding DTD:

```
<NOTE><DATE>January 15th 1993</DATE>
<AUTHOR><FSTNAME>Christian</FSTNAME><LSTNAME>Fluhr</LSTNAME>
</AUTEUR>
<ADDRESSEE><FSTNAME>Dominique</FSTNAME><LSTNAME>Burger
</LSTNAME><FSTNAME>Dominique</FSTNAME><LSTNAME>Béroule
</LSTNAME></ADDRESSEE>
<CONTENT><P>Meeting at Orsay January 20th.</P>
</CONTENT></NOTE>
```

One physical form of this document could be:

```
                    NOTE

                                      January 15th 1993
    ─────────────────────────────────────────────────────
    from: Christian Fluhr           to: Dominique Burger
                                        Dominique Broule


    Meeting at Orsay on January 20th.
```

This supposes that the non variable strings of the note are considered to be given by the formatting procedures. This can also be included in the logical description in SGML. But in this case, the diversity of physical formats is lower.

INFORMATION MANIPULATIONS

If we assume that texts can be obtained in the form of character strings and a standardised coding of the structure, many automatic manipulations can be done. This hypothesis is not very strong because an increasing number of texts can be obtained in their text processing form and the others (if their printing quality is not too poor) can be transformed from image to character by the use of an O.C.R. system.

We will restrict our survey to information acquisition and memorisation. There are many different attitudes to information searching (Rapport du groupe de travail sur le poste de lecteur[1]):

• Very precise information can be searched for to aid decision making. The aim here is to locate, as precisely as possible, all the parts of text in the computer that could be used to make the decision. The work is done in a minimum of time if the system only gives information suitable for the decision (high precision).

• Documents can be browsed quickly to acquire an idea of the subject. They can then be stored for future use. In this case, the user may wish to add comments on the apparent content in order to facilitate a future search of the documents by the same user when the contents will be relevant to making a decision.

• Documents can be read in an exploratory way, without a precise goal, but the user wishes to obtain general information on the field. This mode of reading can be used in Computer Based Training.

• Arriving documents can be sent to people interested in the subject. In this case, the reader just has to declare an interest in a particular subject to be notified if a document arrives. This method is know as information routing.

• Information retrieval can be used to help people writing new texts or updating existing ones. Multi-window environments allow the simultaneous use of a word processor and the search for information. Cut and paste can be used to take parts of the searched texts and to introduce them into the new one. In the case of the updating of a text, a modification in one place can have consequences in others. A retrieval system can be used to extract all the parts of the text that are candidate for a modification.

---

[1] *Rapport du groupe de travail sur le poste du lecteur* can be obtained from Bibliothèque de France, 1 place Valhubert, 75013 Paris France.

TOOLS FOR INFORMATION MANIPULATION

Because of the various means of manipulating information, there are several types of tools that can be used (Debili and al.,1989; Engelen, 1992; Fluhr, 1990; Fluhr, 1991; Fluhr, 1992; Kochanek, 1992).

Full text information retrieval

The full text must be searched in order to obtain the most precise location of information. This is not very easy because the user may look for words that differ from those used by the authors. Even if the same words are used, they may be in a different form (because of plurals, case, conjugation, etc...). Thus, searching with very simple tools is not efficient for a standard user.

It is now possible to obtain quite good results for non specialists in documentation by using retrieval systems that do a linguistic analysis of the text and queries which computes the semantic proximity between the two. In these systems, all the linguistic problems of searching are automatically manage by the computer which processes the query expressed in natural language. Such systems can use terminological databases to infer new words from the original description of what is being searched for. It is also possible to make a translation, like in the EMIR ESPRIT project, where a query in one language can interrogate text in another language (Fluhr, 1990). These systems can compute the semantic proximity between the description of what is being searched for (query) expressed in natural language and the texts in the database which are also in natural language. The result of the search is an ordered list of texts according to an estimation of relevance. A more efficient localisation can be obtain if the document structure is given to the system.

The fact that interrogation in natural language is possible is very important for handicapped people, because it greatly reduces dialogue. For example, one natural language query is equivalent to a strategy of many boolean queries expressed in the very strict computer language found in older information retrieval systems.

Hypertext

A hypertext is the possibility of reading a text in a nonsequential way: The reader can go from one part of the text to another or from one text to another by using links between related texts.

There are many ways of making a hypertext. The first is to automatise links in the paper version of the document. These links can be automatically created from the SGML markups for example. The following can be cited:
- table of contents to the paragraphs,
- cross references to other parts of the document or other documents
- access to figures
- access to notes

Another way of making hypertext links is to manually link parts of texts that provide different aspects of the same object. It is the same problem as cross references but whereas their number is limited in the paper form, they can be far more numerous in the electronic form. Generally links are created according to the supposed intention of users as imagined by the author of the hypertext. It is not possible to imagine all possible kinds of problems that a user may request, so all possible links cannot be established during hypertext construction.

This is why other kinds of hypertext links have been proposed: dynamic hypertext links. These links are dynamically established during the consultation of the text. Users select a part of the text that gives a good idea of what they are looking for and ask the system what parts of the same text or other tests can give information on the same subject. This process uses the same computation of semantic proximity as the full text retrieval system which compares a query in natural language with texts.

Routing information to the right user

Routing information according to the semantic content can be carried out by the same tools as above. Here, semantic proximity is computed between new information and a declaration of interest given previously by the user. Both are in natural language and the semantic comparison can give an estimated degree of interest for each user. If this degree of interest is above a certain limit, the information is sent to the user.

Exploring the content of a text database

A user may wish to know very quickly the content of a textual database. One way is to make conceptual maps that group documents on the same subject. It is then possible to attribute key-words to each cluster of documents to give an idea of their contents.

Another possibility is to show concept graphs representing the main concepts of the database. These concepts are linked with hierarchical semantic relationships. An example of this approach can be seen with the TOPIC [TM] system where the concept graph is constructed by the user and thus represents the user's interests rather than the contents of the database.

A good representation of the content of the database can be obtained by automatically computing the graph from the text database as is done by Systex [1].

[TM] TOPIC is a trademark of Verity, inc, USA.

[1] Systex, Saint Aubin, France.

Here is an example of a part of graph on a patent database on image transmission:

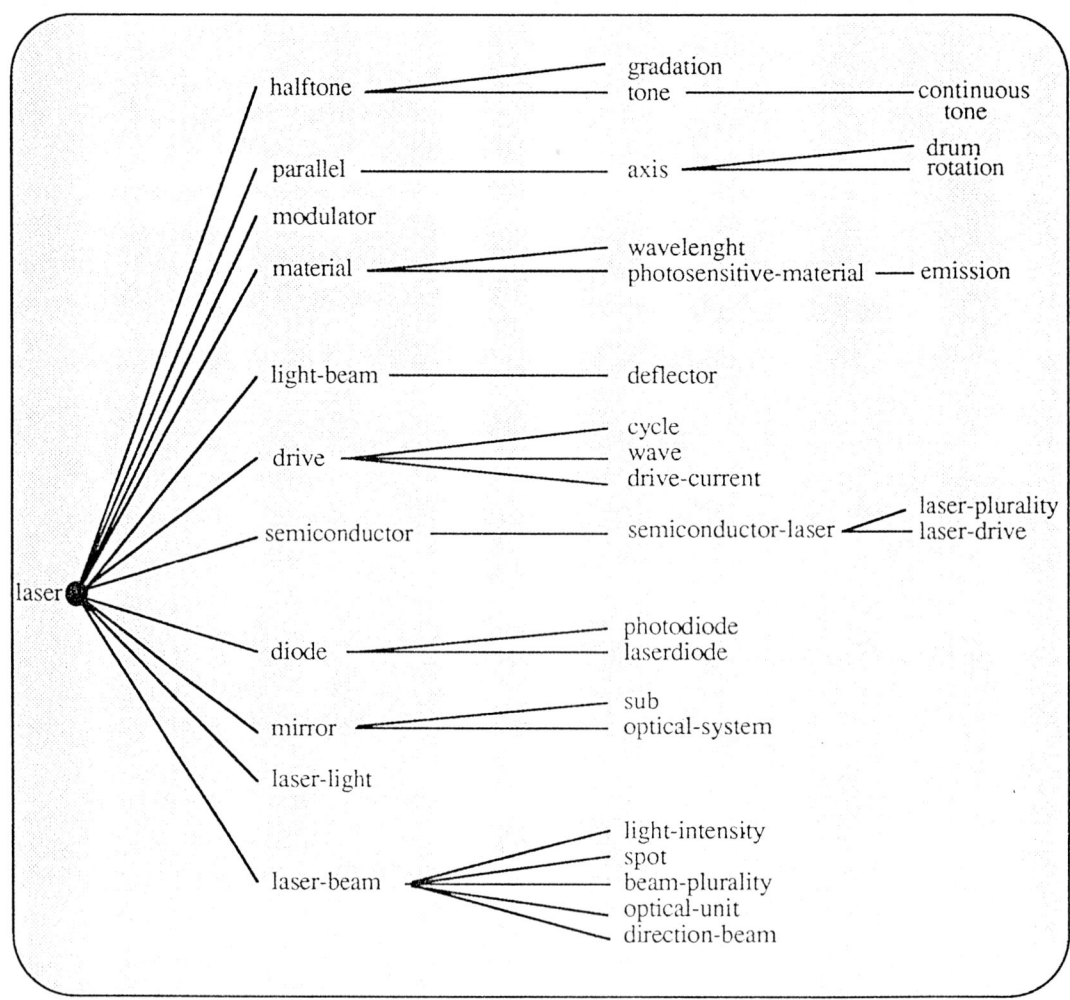

ADAPTABLE HELP TO THE USER

Even if the systems are powerful for searching, it is necessary to offer personalised help to the user. It is very important to know how well users know the domain of the text they are manipulating. This information has a particular influence on the reformulation process which means that the system will not infer the same words from the original query if it knows that the user is a novice or an expert in the domain.

Explanations of what can be done in a particular situation will not be given with the same words if the user is a secretary or an engineer. The system can also detect incoherences in the user's behaviour and suggest learning aspects of the system that do not seem to be understood.

Information about the user may be obtained directly by asking the user, and in addition, the help system may have its own senses to observe the user's behaviour.

Techniques invented for the Intelligent Computer Training systems can be used for this. These systems, like STARGUIDE ™ (Claes, 1988), are based on a filtering of the dialogue between the user and the application. The training or help system can observe the dialogue, then it can:
• take the initiative of transforming the user input into another input to the application, either to correct erroneous inputs or to convert adapted input for a particular user into the standard input.
• transform the application output into another form or add an explanation.
• demonstrate functions of the application by sending commands to it.
• ask the user for explanations.

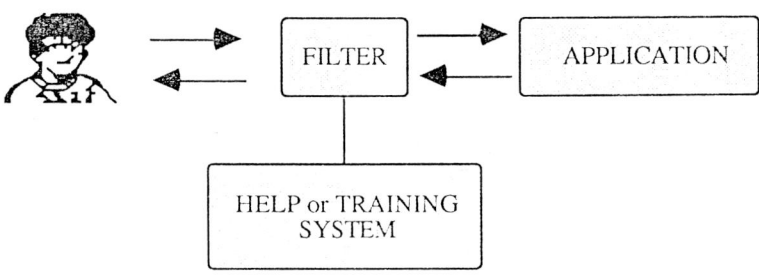

This kind of architecture can also be used for adapting standard application interfaces to a particular user population. For example, this architecture can be used to capture dialogue between an application and a GUI environment (Graphic User Interface) allowing the adaptation of dialogue to people who cannot use graphic interfaces like the blind. Because the filtering system can do what it wants with the output of the application - transform it and forward it to the interface or transform it and pilot its own interface - it is able to completely mask the standard interface and adapt it to a completely different form. On the other hand, the commands sent by the user can be simplified if the user only uses some aspects of the application. The filtering system can translate the simplified commands into the standard ones.

™ Starguide is a trademark of Bull, marketed by A6, Evry, France.

This type of functionality is also of interest for general users in problems of interface inhomogeneity. This is the case for CD-ROMs where each CD publisher uses different interfaces. It is very difficult for people who question various disks to commute from one interface to another. If it was possible to filter the dialogue, it would be possible to give an homogeneous interface for all the disks that have the same type of access. It would be necessary to build an adaptation of dialogue to the standard interface for each disk by the use of the filter.

CONCLUSION

Some possible uses of paper documents can no longer be used with electronic documents. For example the global view of a book or the fast reading of pages to locate the right page. This kind of information access is precisely what the blind cannot do. The new way of reading proposed by electronic documents improves blind peoples chances because they can use the computer in the same way as sighted people.

The main problem remaining originates in the increasing use of graphic interfaces. This kind of interface enables sighted people to use the computer faster.

It is therefore necessary to transform the interface for blind people into speech synthesis or a braille display. Techniques used with standard interfaces (reading of output buffer) are not applicable because buffers of GUI contain bitmaps and not characters. Filtering techniques can solve this problem. They can adapt dialogue with applications without accessing the code of the application, simply by capturing and rerouting messages exchanged between the interface object and the application. This technique can also be used to provide help to particular categories of users and to train users to get the best from the application. This in very important in reading applications particularly for the blind.

All these techniques exist separately, but at this moment in time, no one has integrated them into a single system. We can hope that projects initiated by the European Community such as TIDE (Technology Initiative for Disabled and Elderly) or national programs can help research teams and companies to reach this goal.

REFERENCES

Claes G., Ounis O., Razoarivelo Z., Salembier P. & Sridharan M. (1988), STARGUIDE, A generator for self tutorials, In *Proceedings of the RIAO Conference*, MIT Cambridge, march 1988, p.259-274.

Danish Standards Association (1991), *SGML-ODA, Présentation des concepts et comparaison fonctionnelle*. Collection AFNOR Technique, 104 p.

Debili F., Fluhr C. & Radasoa P. (1989), Information processing and management, About reformulation in *full text IRS*, Vol. 25, N° 6, p.647-657.

Engelen J. & Baldewuns J. (1992), Digital Information distribution for the reading impaired: From daily newspaper to whole libraries, In *Proceedings of the 3rd International Conference on Computers for handicapped persons*, Vienna, 7-9 July 1992, p.144-149.

Fluhr C. (1990), Multilingual access to full-text databases, In *Proceedings of the International Artificial Intelligence Symposium*, november 14-16, 1990, Nagoya, Japan, p.107-110.

Fluhr C. (1990), Dynamic Hypertext links, In *Proceedings of the JIPDEC-CID International Symposium on Trends of Intelligent Hypermedia*, Tokyo, 25-26 October 1990, p.81-87.

Fluhr C. & Machard C. (1991),Gateways "intelligents", In *Bringing down the Barriers to Information Transfer*, AGARD Conference Proceedings, n°505, Neuilly France: ed. AGARD, p.21-28.

Fluhr C. (1992), Le traitement du langage naturel dans la recherhe d'information documentaire, in Interfaces intelligentes dans l'information scientifique et technique, In *proceedings of INRIA Seminar*, Klingenthal, 18-22 mai 1992.

Kochanek D. (1992), A hypertext system for The Blind newspaper reader, In *proceedings of 3rd International Conference on Computers for handicapped persons*, Vienna, 7-9 July 1992, p.285-293.

Van Herwijnen E. (1990), *Practical SGML*, Dordrecht: Kluwer Academic Publishers, 307 p.

Résumé

De plus en plus fréquemment les documents sont archivés et présentés au lecteur sur support informatisé, de sorte que de nouvelles méthodes de consultation doivent être mises au point pour remplacer les méthodes traditionnelles de lecture des documents sur papier. Cet article décrit les nouveaux besoins et les nouveaux outils logiciels liés à la recherche d'information. Le principe de ces outils repose sur l'analyse du contenu sous forme de chaîne de caractères et de la structure des textes. Ils permettent donc d'accéder au sens indépendamment de la forme même.

Les standards de codage des documents structurés sont présentés. Différentes méthodes d'interrogation des documents sont passées en revue ainsi que des logiciels d'accès. La nécessité de personnaliser les systèmes d'accès, et en particulier les possibilités d'adaptation pour les personnes aveugles sont également discutées.

Colloques **INSERM**
ISSN 0768-3154

Other *Colloques* published as co-editions by John Libbey Eurotext and INSERM

153 Hormones and Cell Regulation (11th European Symposium). *Hormones et Régulation Cellulaire (11e Symposium Européen).*
Edited by J. Nunez and J.E. Dumont.
ISBN : John Libbey Eurotext 0 86196 104 8
INSERM 2 85598 324 X

158 Biochemistry and Physiopathology of Platelet Membrane. *Biochimie et Physiopathologie de la Membrane Plaquettaire.*
Edited by G. Marguerie and R.F.A. Zwaal.
ISBN : John Libbey Eurotext 0 86196 114 5
INSERM 2 85598 345 2

162 The Inhibitors of Hematopoiesis. *Les Inhibiteurs de l'Hématopoïèse.*
Edited by A. Najman, M. Guignon, N.C. Gorin and J.Y. Mary.
ISBN : John Libbey Eurotext 0 86196 125 0
INSERM 2 85598 340 1

164 Liver Cells and Drugs. *Cellules Hépatiques et Médicaments.*
Edited by A. Guillouzo.
ISBN : John Libbey Eurotext 0 86196 128 5
INSERM 2 85598 341 X

165 Hormones and Cell Regulation (12th European Symposium). *Hormones et Régulation Cellulaire (12e Symposium Européen).*
Edited by J. Nunez, J.E. Dumont and E. Carafoli.
ISBN : John Libbey Eurotext 0 86196 133 1
INSERM 2 85598 347 9

167 Sleep Disorders and Respiration. *Les Evénements Respiratoires du Sommeil.*
Edited by P. Lévi-Valensi and D. Duron.
ISBN : John Libbey Eurotext 0 86196 127 7
INSERM 2 85598 344 4

169 Neo-Adjuvant Chemotherapy. *Chimiothérapie Néo-Adjuvante.*
Edited by C. Jacquillat, M. Weil, D. Khayat.
ISBN : John Libbey Eurotext 0 86196 150 1
INSERM 2 85598 349 5

171 Structure and Functions of the Cytoskeleton. *La Structure et les Fonctions du Cytosquelette.*
Edited by B.A.F. Rousset.
ISBN : John Libbey Eurotext 0 86196 149 8
INSERM 2 85598 351 7

Colloques INSERM
ISSN 0768-3154

172 The Langerhans Cell. *La Cellule de Langerhans.*
Edited by J. Thivolet, D. Schmitt.
ISBN : John Libbey Eurotext 0 86196 181 1
INSERM 2 85598 352 5

173 Cellular and Molecular Aspects of Glucuronidation. *Aspects Cellulaires et Moléculaires de la Glucuronoconjugaison.*
Edited by G. Siest, J. Magdalou, B. Burchell
ISBN : John Libbey Eurotext 0 86196 182 X
INSERM 2 85598 353 3

174 Second Forum on Peptides. *Deuxième Forum Peptides.*
Edited by A. Aubry, M. Marraud, B. Vitoux
ISBN : John Libbey Eurotext 0 86196 151 X
INSERM 2 85598 354 1

176 Hormones and Cell Regulation (13th European Symposium). *Hormones et Régulation Cellulaire (13e Symposium Européen).*
Edited by J. Nunez, J.E. Dumont, R. Denton
ISBN : John Libbey Eurotext 0 86196 183 8
INSERM 2 85598 356 8

179 Lymphokine Receptors Interactions. *Interactions Lymphokines-recepteurs.*
Edited by D. Fradelizi, J. Bertoglio
ISBN : John Libbey Eurotext 0 86196 148 X
INSERM 2 85598 359 2

191 Anticancer Drugs (1st International Interface of Clinical and Laboratory responses to anticancer drugs). *Médicaments anticancéreux (1re Confrontation internationale des réponses cliniques et expérimentales aux médicaments anticancéreux).*
Edited by H. Tapiero, J. Robert, T.J. Lampidis
ISBN : John Libbey Eurotext 0 86196 223 0
INSERM 2 85598 393 2

193 Living in the Cold (2nd International Symposium). *La Vie au Froid (2e Symposium International).*
Edited by A. Malan, B. Canguilhem
ISBN : John Libbey Eurotext 0 86196 234 9
INSERM 2 85598 395 9

Colloques INSERM
ISSN 0768-3154

194 Progress in Hepatitis B Immunization. *La Vaccination contre l'épatite B.*
Edited by P. Coursaget, M.J. Tong
ISBN : John Libbey Eurotext 0 86196 249 4
INSERM 2 85598 396 7

196 Treatment Strategy in Hodgkin's Disease. *Stratégie dans la maladie de Hodgkin.*
Edited by P. Sommers, M. Henry-Amar,
J.H. Meezwaldt, P. Carde
ISBN : John Libbey Eurotext 0 86196 226 5
INSERM 2 85598 398 3

198 Hormones and Cell Regulation (14th European Symposium). *Hormones et Régulation Cellulaire (14e Symposium Européen).*
Edited by J. Nunez, J.E. Dumont
ISBN : John Libbey Eurotext 0 86196 229 X
INSERM 2 85598 400 9

199 Placental Communications : Biochemical, Morphological and Cellular Aspects. *Communications placentaires : aspects biochimique, morphologique et cellulaire.*
Edited by L. Cedard, E. Alsat, J.C. Challier,
G. Chaouat, A. Malassiné
ISBN : John Libbey Eurotext 0 86196 227 3
INSERM 2 85598 401 7

204 Pharmacologie Clinique : Actualités et Perspectives. (6e Rencontres Nationales de Pharmacologie clinique).
Edited by J.P. Boissel, C. Caulin, M. Teule
ISBN : John Libbey Eurotext 0 86196 225 7
INSERM 2 85598 454 8

205 Recent Trends in Clinical Pharmacology (6th National Meeting of Clinical Pharmacology).
Edited by J.P. Boissel, C. Caulin, M. Teule
ISBN : John Libbey Eurotext 0 86196 256 7
INSERM 2 85598 455 6

206 Platelet Immunology : Fundamental and Clinical Aspects. *Immunologie plaquettaire : aspects fondamentaux et cliniques.*
Edited by C. Kaplan-Gouet, N. Schlegel,
Ch. Salmon, J. McGregor
ISBN : John Libbey Eurotext 0 86196 285 0
INSERM 2 85598 439 4

Colloques INSERM
ISSN 0768-3154

207 Thyroperoxidase and Thyroid Autoimmunity.
Thyroperoxydase et auto-immunité thyroïdienne.
Edited by P. Carayon, T. Ruf
ISBN : John Libbey Eurotext 0 86196 277 X
    INSERM 2 85598 440 8

208 Vasopressin. *Vasopressine.*
Edited by S. Jard, R. Jamison
ISBN : John Libbey Eurotext 0 86196 288 5
    INSERM 2 85598 441 6

210 Hormones and Cell Regulation (15th European Symposium). *Hormones et Régulation Cellulaire (15ᵉ Symposium Européen).*
Edited by J.E. Dumont, J. Nunez, R.J.B. King
ISBN : John Libbey Eurotext 0 86196 279 6
    INSERM 2 85598 443 2

211 Medullary Thyroid Carcinoma. *Cancer Médullaire de la Thyroïde.*
Edited by C. Calmettes, J.M. Guliana
ISBN : John Libbey Eurotext 0 86196 287 7
    INSERM 2 85598 440 0

212 Cellular and Molecular Biology of the Materno-Fetal Relationship. *Biologie cellulaire et moléculaire de la relation materno-fœtale.*
Edited by G. Chaouat, J. Mowbray
ISBN : John Libbey Eurotext 0 86196 909 1
    INSERM 2 85598 445 9

215 Aldosterone. Fundamental Aspects.
Aspects fondamentaux.
Edited by J.P. Bonvalet, N. Farman, M. Lombes, M.E. Rafestin-Oblin
ISBN : John Libbey Eurotext 0 86196 302 4
    INSERM 2 85598 482 3

216 Cellular and Molecular Aspects of Cirrhosis.
Aspects cellulaires et moléculaires de la cirrhose.
Edited by B. Clément, A. Guillouzo
ISBN : John Libbey Eurotext 0 86196 342 3
    INSERM 2 85598 483 1

217 Sleep and Cardiorespiratory Control. *Sommeil et contrôle cardio-respiratoire.*
Edited by C. Gaultier, P. Escourrou, L. Curzi-Dascalora
ISBN : John Libbey Eurotext 0 86196 307 5
    INSERM 2 85598 484 X

Colloques INSERM
ISSN 0768-3154

218 Genetic Hypertension. *Hypertension génétique.*
Edited by J. Sassard
ISBN : John Libbey Eurotext 0 86196 313 X
INSERM 2 85598 485 8

219 Human Gene Transfer. *Transfert de gènes chez l'homme.*
Edited by O. Cohen-Haguenauer, M. Boiron
ISBN : John Libbey Eurotext 0 86196 301 6
INSERM 2 85598 497 1

221 Structures and Functions of Retinal Proteins. *Structures et fonctions des rétino-protéines.*
Edited by J.L. Rigaud
ISBN : John Libbey Eurotext 0 86196 355 5
INSERM 2 85598 509 9

222 Cellular and Molecular Biology of the Adrenal Cortex. *Biologie cellulaire et moléculaire du cortex surrénal.*
Edited by J.M. Saez, A.C. Brownic, A. Capponi, E.M. Chambaz, F. Mantero
ISBN : John Libbey Eurotext 0 86196 362 8
INSERM 2 85598 510 2

223 Mechanisms and Control of Emesis. *Mécanismes et contrôle du vomissement.*
Edited by A.L. Bianchi, L. Grélot, A.D. Miller, G.L. King
ISBN : John Libbey Eurotext 0 86196 363 6
INSERM 2 85598 511 0

224 High Pressure and Biotechnology. *Haute pression et biotechnologie.*
Edited by C. Balny, R. Hayashi, K. Heremans, P. Masson
ISBN : John Libbey Eurotext 0 86196 363 6
INSERM 2 85598 512 9

Free service for visually handicapped readers
Service gratuit pour les lecteurs handicapés de la vue

People who have difficulty in reading this book can order the ascii file of the texts (3" 1/2 disk) free of charge by filling in the form below and sending it to:

Les personnes ne pouvant lire ce livre peuvent commander la version ascii des textes sur disquette 3"1/2 en remplissant le bon de commande ci-dessous et en le retournant à :

Secrétariat ANPEA-SETAA
12 bis, rue Picpus
75012 Paris - France

Only original order forms will be accepted - Please no photocopy

Merci d'utiliser l'original du bon de commande - Photocopie non acceptée

---

Please send me a copy of the Conference Proceedings ascii file
"Non-Visual Human-Computer Interactions" (Paris,1993)

Merci de m'adresser une copie du fichier ascii des Actes du Colloque
"Communication non-Visuelle Homme-Ordinateur" *(Paris,1993)*

Name/Nom : ....
Organisation/Organisme: ....
....
Address/ Adresse : ....
....
City/Ville : ....
....
Country/ Pays : ....Postal code/ Code postal................

LOUIS-JEAN
avenue d'Embrun, 05003 GAP cedex
Tél. : 92.53.17.00
Dépôt légal : 217 — Mars 1993
Imprimé en France